The Purpose of This Book

My dream for this book is to reach one person at a time and help them in some way. I wrote this book about my learning disability, but this is for anyone who has his or her own special challenge. In this book I tell you about my struggles and accomplishments as a child and an adult with Dyslexia, with the hope that it will give you the strength and encouragement to help yourself or a loved one. It has been a long road, but I wouldn't change a thing. I am the person I am today because of all the mountains and valleys I have conquered. I strongly urge you to read this book and apply it to your life. Don't ever give up on your dreams and always believe in yourself.

Thought you might find this book helpful. This man spoke at Jordan's school. His story awesome.

FOREWORD

Ann Phillips, Ph.D., L.P.C.
Coordinator, Disabled Student Services
State University of West Georgia

I first met Rob when he became a student at West Georgia College. He had an engaging smile and a great air about him. He also had a learning disability – Dyslexia. Together, Rob and I worked to find ways for him to be a successful student. At the time, West Georgia College offered no provisions for accommodating learning-disabled students. Seven long years and many accommodations later, Rob graduated from West Georgia College (now the State University of West Georgia) with a B.F.A., with a focus on Graphic Design. The invaluable legacy he left behind was that the "Office of Disabled Student Services" now covered learning disabilities in addition to physical disabilities. It provides a more knowledgeable and experienced staff to address the needs of learning disabled students. Due to Rob's pioneering spirit and courage, over two-hundred learning-disabled students are now receiving accommodations that allow them to be successful at the State University of West Georgia.

I am proud of what Rob has accomplished and honored to have worked with him. Over the years, we shared joy and frustration, ups and downs. More than anything, we shared the conviction that Rob would and could graduate from college. I have watched him grow and develop into one whose life is devoted to helping others. The value of the precedents he left behind for learning disabled students is incalculable. Many others would not have been given a chance and are now proudly college graduates. Thanks, Rob, for sharing your exciting adventure with me and now with others.

Table of Contents

Part 1: The 100 Year Goal

CHAPTER 1

Part 2: The Path to Success

CHAPTER 2

CHAPTER 3

CHAPTER 4

Part 3: Getting What You Need

Acknowledgements

Many people have helped me over the years including teachers, counselors and friends. However, I particularly want to acknowledge the people who helped me the most, my family. The support, love and commitment of my family are expressed early on in this book. Because of them, I have achieved much for which I am proud. Mom, Dad, my brother, Lon and my sister, Natalie each gave me a unique and priceless gift. My Aunt Margianna Langston, a writer in Atlanta, Georgia was of special assistance in writing and researching this book. She has taken my words and put them to paper, helping me to share my message.

Mom was my first advocate in learning and in life, and she taught me to be an advocate for myself. She was by my side every step of the way, protecting my self-esteem and getting me what I needed to learn. I'm sure she experienced frustrations and tears that I knew nothing about at the time, but she was determined that nothing would stop me. She went through the discomfort of being the "squeaky wheel" at school in order to get me what I needed to learn.

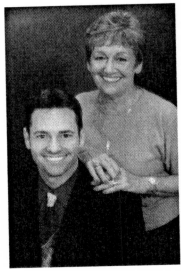

She had no special training in learning disabilities. It simply was her mission to foster happy, loving, responsible children. No one could ever convince her I was dumb. She always operated on the premise that her son was smart at home, but failing in school; therefore there must be something wrong with the school. Mom is truly my hero.

Dad was my role model and example. His love and example of living were a source of great strength to me. He taught me about commitment and about caring. Dad always supported me, and at times I felt that he even admired me. I am proud of him as well, not only because he was a successful businessman and loving father, but also for the person he is and the inspiration and support he has always given to me.

Lon, my brother is three years older and also has dyslexia. His did not show up as early as mine or was as extreme a form. Throughout school he tested very high for intelligence, but had trouble reading. As older siblings often do, Lon paved the road for me. In fourth grade they called Mom in for a conference and said that Lon was not passing, although he was in the remedial group. Mom sat him down and talked to him about why he wasn't doing well. He told her that he was in the lowest group, but all his friends were in the highest group. He knew he could do better if he was with his friends. Mom went to school and asked them to move Lon into the group with his friends, although the school did not recommend the move, she persisted until they agreed. She even signed a waiver saying she would take responsibility if Lon could not do the work. Lon started making C's in his new class. I am very grateful to Lon and very proud of him. He graduated from college with a business degree and is now a successful businessman with a wonderful wife and two beautiful daughters. Because of his open communication with my mom, she was able to understand the problem and help him in his work and gain self-esteem.

My younger sister, Natalie, holds a special place in my heart. She is three years younger than me, and we were in high school and college at the same time. I was her buddy and protector, but she was also mine. When people thought I was stupid, or said mean things about me, she came immediately to my defense. Natalie never had any trouble learning, but she was generous in helping me with my lessons by reading to me in the car on the way to school or at night.

Natalie taught me a lot about truth and determination. She may have had setbacks in her own life, but she never lost the desire to succeed. She still has a tremendous determination to get what she wants out of life. Her support and compassion continue to be an inspiration to me.

My deepest thanks go to my wife Jeannette who has been beside me every step of the way in writing this book. She has supported my dream to make a difference for the children. She has been willing to risk everything for me to do this work. She waited four years for our marriage to occur so I could get my business off the ground. Then she waited two more years for our home, the one we took a second mortgage out on so I could finish writing this book. She was even ready to sell our home so we could generate the seed money to start the For the Children Foundation.

I also want to thank my precious daughter Noble. She is my strength and resolve. I look at Noble and I'm proud of what I am trying to do and I'm proud of what this book is trying to do. This book and the foundation are my small attempts to make life a little better for my little girl and all children. She symbolizes everything that I am working for.

Dyslexia is an inherited condition and we have no way of knowing if she has it. We had a scare shortly after she was born; she failed a hearing test in her right ear. Because my mother taught me how to be an advocate, I was able to get my daughter the proper tests and her hearing is fine. From day one I have been fighting for her, and always will.

In my experience throughout my educational career, I have found that the teachers' stories I share in this book fall into three categories. The first category is teachers who start out with some struggle but then go on to be academic leaders, second is pioneering teachers, and third is character-building teachers. All the stories share their own struggle and success and how it's extremely hard to achieve great success without strengthening your "overcoming-obstacle muscles." The hopefulness about all my stories of struggle is they seem to always have a silver lining.

Part 1: The 100 Year Goal

CHAPTER 1

An Able Person with a Learning Disability

I'm Rob Langston and I have dyslexia.

It wasn't always easy for me to introduce myself that way. For much of my life, I struggled to feel normal, to survive in school, to be accepted by my friends, and to stay out of trouble. I lied, cheated, and tried to hide my disability. When I was in second grade, they tested my IQ at 84. I entered college reading at the fifth grade level. There were times when I didn't know if I'd make it. But with the help of my family, friends, and some very special educators like Dr. Ann Phillips, I not only survived but also thrived. I earned a college degree, and was hired by a major corporation to speak to people across the country about learning disabilities. Each year I conduct seminars on success for an international organization of over 8,000 CEO's of companies doing more than $175 billion in sales.

I get up every morning of my life and do what I love doing more than anything else and I get paid to do it. I've talked to hundreds of thousands of parents, students, and teachers about how to keep your self-esteem intact and succeed beyond your wildest dreams, even when you have what people call a disability.

My disability taught me things about myself, about life, and about success that were priceless. I don't think I could have learned them any other way. One of the things I learned is that when you succeed, the first thing you have to do is reach out to others and share what you know to help them. That's why I'm writing this book.

I'll talk about how my mom and I discovered my particular learning style and learned to support the educational system in giving me what I needed in order to succeed. I'll tell you what those needs were, and how best to get them accommodated today. Most importantly, I'll present some principles for success and self esteem that anyone can use to achieve their goals and dreams in life, and to make the contributions that they are here to make.

This book is for people with disabilities, for their teachers and loved ones, and also for anyone who wants to succeed based on being a valuable, worthwhile person, regardless of their circumstances. The principles for thriving despite a disability are also principles for everyone to live by. They've empowered me to succeed as a person, as a student, and as a businessman. They will empower you to discover that who you really are is a valuable person, and to find your own way in all areas of life.

The Attitude for Success

Several years ago, I attended the national convention of the Association for Learning Disabilities of America. The speaker asked the audience, which was comprised mainly of learning disabled individuals, to give words that describe learning disabilities. About thirty words were thrown out, including "dumb," "lazy," "stupid," "retarded," "slow," "quiet," "problems," "inadequate," "damaged," and "abnormal."

That was the participants' perception of themselves! If we are calling ourselves these things, why should anyone else call us something different? Unfortunately, many people with learning disabilities, including children, know nothing else. This has been their reality.

My first advice to anyone labeled in these ways is to STOP. Rethink. Change your self-description from "learning disabled" to "learning abled." Today I still read at the seventh grade level, but I am an extremely "able" speaker, so able that I can make my living that way! I can't multiply, but I am a bright, creative person. It is difficult for me to put my thoughts on paper, but I am writing a book. I am "able" enough to be appointed to the State Advisory Panel for Special Education with board members from the academic and political communities. My fellow panel members include the Director of Special Education for the state of Georgia along with many university professors. Highly educated college, high school and elementary school administrators seek my advice concerning programs for special students.

I am able and so are you. It's important to think that way, and to talk that way to yourself and to others.

When I speak to groups about being an able person, I love to tell this story. After I graduated from college I went out and bought a sports car. I thought that's what 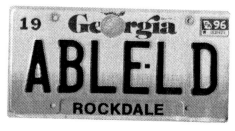 you did when you started making money. It was a shiny red 300 ZX twin turbo, 300 horsepower, with black leather interior. I went over to the Department of Motor Vehicles to get a special tag: ABLE-LD. To me, that meant that I was an able person with a learning disability, but other people didn't necessarily see it that way. They didn't get it. I'd watch them in my rear view mirror, squinting to read that tag, trying to figure out what it meant. And I would think to myself, 'they look just like me, trying to figure out what's written on a piece of paper!'

It was important for me to get that tag, to tell the world that I was an able person. It was a sign of self-esteem, and that's been the most important thing to my success as a student, as a businessman, and as a person.

What it Takes to Succeed

To many people, the terms "learning disabled," and "success" don't go together. The perception is that if you're learning disabled, you can't be successful. But my experience is just the opposite. In fact, I've learned most of what I know, including what it takes to be a success, by living with my disability and not letting it stop me. I've learned what it takes to succeed, whether or not you have a disability, and in the process I've found myself.

What makes people successful? In this book, I'll talk about the principles that emerged out of my journey, so you can see how you can use them to create success in your own life. Here are a few of them:

1. Let people support you.

I became an advocate for myself, and then for other people with disabilities. I watched my mother as an advocate for me when I was growing up, and I took what she taught me and taught it to other people.

2. Communicate.

My mother wouldn't have known what to do for me if I hadn't told her the truth about my disability. We made a quantum leap the moment I said to her, after doing poorly on a test, "Mom, I can't write what I know."

3. Help others with what you've learned.

I may have received my college degree, and probably would have been a success in some business, even if I hadn't become an advocate for people with learning disabilities. On the other hand, I might not have experienced the satisfaction that I have today. Every day I get up and give away all the good things that have come to me, which just brings more good things, and good feelings and good relationships back to me.

4. Focus on your goals.

Everyday my mom focused on the question: How is my child going to learn in school today? She was not a professional educator, but she learned what she needed to learn, and spoke to whomever she had to speak to, and said whatever she had to say so that I could make full use of my day in school. Focus on where you're going, and focus on you gifts instead of your disabilities.

5. Keep your self-esteem strong.

I have a controversial stance on self-esteem. I believe that you can succeed in life without knowing reading, writing, and arithmetic, but you can't succeed without self-esteem. My mother's first concern when I was growing up was to preserve my self-esteem in the midst of situations that looked as if they might destroy it. When I became an advocate for myself, I had the advantage of strong self-esteem. It's your most priceless possession.

6. Remember that everyone is different.

We are all unique human beings, and we each have our own particular way of learning. My greatest blessing was discovering that I wasn't dumb, as some people had assumed. I just had my own style of learning, of taking in and processing information. When that learning style could be accommodated, it was clear that I had above average intelligence. That opened up a whole new world for me.

There are other principles for thriving and succeeding with a disability, and we'll discuss them in the course of this book, but these are the ones to keep in mind as you go through this guide.

Breaking Through Obstacles

We all encounter obstacles in life. Sometimes these obstacles are society's problems such as crime, poverty, and violence and sometimes they are more personal. Sometimes they are big and sometimes they are small. But if we are human beings, we will encounter obstacles. That is our chance to grow.

I spent many miserable years as a "handicapped" child. That experience taught me how to deal with obstacles, as well as how not to deal with them. I'll never forget that day in 8th grade when I misspelled my middle name. I wrote "Willaim" instead of "William." It was a common mistake for someone with dyslexia, but my 8th grade teacher ridiculed me. He pointed out my error and said to the class, "I don't know how any student can get to the 8th grade without knowing how to spell his own name." The class laughed. I forced a half smile and sank lower into my chair, trying to look unaffected. Neither he nor the other students knew how humiliated I felt.

Many years later, I was inducted into that school's Teachers' Hall of Fame for my work in helping children with learning disabilities. That same 8th grade teacher, now the Vice-Principal, was on the selection committee. He graciously and enthusiastically congratulated me on my achievements. It was clear that he had no idea of the pain he had unintentionally caused me.

There are two lessons here. One is to be careful what you say to children, because they are listening. The other is, that no matter how painful an obstacle is, it can be overcome.

The challenge was overcoming an off-handed remark. The silver lining was that this teacher is now what I consider one of the top ten most influential teachers in my life.

As my eighth grade year progressed this teacher gave me the skills that literally kick-started my attitude about overcoming obstacles. This has been one of the strongest tools in my life. That year became the turning point for which the rest of my life has been measured. I was chosen to be in a new program that year incorporating classroom learning with outdoor learning called SOAR. The

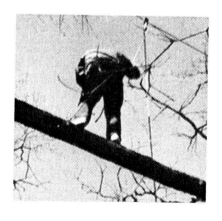
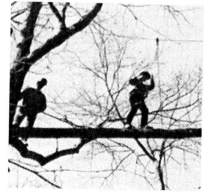

program of outdoor learning required the participants to complete an incredible ropes course the school had built that summer. Today this program is usually associated with Project Adventure (www.pa.org).

Over the next years of my life, the same teacher that had unknowingly wounded me, also taught me to overcome mental and physical obstacles.

At that time, I thought it was impossible. I tell this story today to CEOs about looking down from 30 feet in the air and having to complete some of the scarriest challenges of my life. Ironically, it was always this teacher at the other end of my rope. He was my lifeline, shouting encouragement and catching me if ever I fell. I have found that almost every teacher that's part of a story of struggle in this book, can be attributed with 90% positive growth in my life. This is compared to only a 10% negative impact. I would like to also point out that the negative impact almost always came prior to the teacher and I getting to know one another. The shot fired for not knowing how to spell my name came during the first week of one of the greatest personal growth years of my life led by, you guessed it, my eighth grade teacher.

At the end of my talks to students and teachers, I do a demonstration of breaking through obstacles. I place two cinderblocks on the floor, and then balance between them two wood boards measuring one foot by one foot by one inch. I prepare myself with breathing and concentration, and then I break the boards with my hand.

This involves practice and a lot of focus. Sometimes people think I'm focusing on the boards I'm going to break. Nothing could be farther from the truth! If I focused on those boards, on the obstacles, my hand and wrist

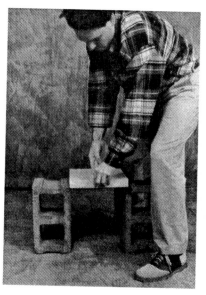
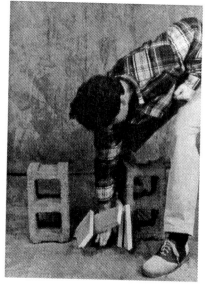

would go flying into a million pieces. No, I focus on the floor. I put my attention on the goal, on the solution, on the place I'm going to be when I've broken through the obstacles. Then I simply thrust my hand down to where I'm aiming, at the floor, and it goes effortlessly through the obstacles, the boards.

When you break through obstacles, you have to focus on the positive, not the negative. If you focus on getting what you want, you will pass through the obstacles and only notice them when you are on the other side and have already succeeded past them.

Make the Journey Positive

For many years, I only focused on my problem, on my disability. However, when I discovered that I was smart and that I just learned differently from other people, I stopped doing that. I became a success in my own mind, and I started being a success in school. The transformation from "a learning disabled" to "an able person" began at that moment for me. When I stopped focusing on the disability and started focusing on the fact that I was smart, I began to succeed.

There were many painful moments during my school years and many pleasurable ones. Looking back from where I am now, it's hard to characterize any of those moments as "good" or "bad." Each of them was "character-building," in that it made me what I am today. I do not regret any of them, because every experience helped me grow and mold my character.

It has been a long road full of curves, bends, detours and dead-ends, but every bend taught me to let go of self-doubt and limitations and led me toward the path of self-fulfillment. My creativity, my talents, and my self-esteem are now free to be expressed. This is happiness. And this is success.

My 100-Year Vision

My 100-year goal is to change the education system, as we know it today. Today, it is generally believed that we only teach about 30% of our children effectively. The reason for this is that we test them primarily on how they read and write, but only about 30% of them learn this way. We completely ignore auditory, visual, kinesthetic, and other modes of learning.

Everyone has a different learning style. My goal is find out what each student's learning style is and honor it so that every child has a chance to learn in school. We have to teach children the way they learn, not the way we've always taught in the past just because, "that's the way it has always been done."

In schools of education, we teach teachers to prepare lesson plans and follow them, but not every student moves at the same pace, or in the same direction. Most children are not going to be where the lesson plan wants them to be, on the day when the lesson plan wants them to be there. Most people simply don't fit into that mold.

I have learned through my own experience and through the work I do that if you don't make it in education, it becomes highly likely that you won't make it in life or in society. We will see in another chapter what happens to people who don't make it in education, and what happens to our society when those people don't make it. Instead of contributing to society, they take and take and take. Anything we invest in helping them succeed in school is money, time, and energy well spent.

My vision for the education system is that it becomes an environment of acceptance, an environment in which it is okay to be different, okay to learn differently, and okay to tell the truth and ask for help. This is the way we develop "lifelong learners," and I believe that lifelong learning should be the goal of the education system.

I am not an expert in the science of education; I do not have advanced educational degrees. I know very little about medical procedures or therapies that diagnose or cure learning disabilities. This book is about what worked for me. I can only show my own results and the path that led me to success. Everyone with learning disabilities must discover his or her own way to being a happy, productive citizen. My hope is that this book will inspire you to do just that.

Part II: The Path to Success

CHAPTER 2

Learning How I Learned: Elementary and Middle School

I learned about my learning disability through trial and error, which meant going to school, having trouble, allowing my mother to be an advocate for me, and following her lead in finding solutions. In elementary school, most of our time was spent defining the problem and working our way toward common sense solutions.

High Hopes

Like many five year-olds, I thought I was a "big boy" when I went to kindergarten. The day following Labor Day, I jumped out of bed, dressed in my new long pants, gathered my Scooby Doo lunch box, and impatiently waited at the front door for my mother to take me to my first day of school. I was an outgoing, gregarious kid and had no fear of leaving my mother.

When we arrived at the kindergarten room, I smiled and said "Hi" to the nice "older" ladies, my teachers who were fresh out of college. They were kind to me and to the rest of the class. We colored, made music with wooden instruments, ate lunch as a group in the cafeteria, and took naps on our special mats. My favorite activity was cookies and milk time. I excelled at this.

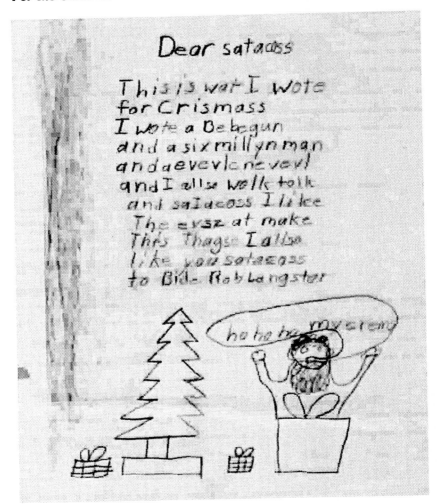

Dear Santa Claus
This is what I want
for Christmas
I want a Bebe gun
and a six million dollar man
and an evil kenevil
and I also want walkie talkies
and santa claus I like
the elves that make
these things. I also
like you santa claus
to By Rob Langston

The months passed and I was cutting, pasting and eating glue with the best of them. Life was good. School really lived up to my expectations. At the end of the year, my teacher told my mother and me, "Rob is 100% ready for the first grade." With the confidence of a six-year-old, I wondered if first grade was ready for me.

The summer passed slowly, as it always does when you are waiting for a special event, and going to the first grade was a big event for me. I had visions of reading stories to my family, counting my own money, tying my shoelaces, and all the other things that "big boys" do. Finally the day arrived. As a veteran of kindergarten, I confidently slung my book bag over my left shoulder, carried my lunch box in my right hand and headed off to the first grade.

Again, the teacher greeted me warmly and said she was glad I was in her class. I was happy, too. But it did not take long to see that things were different in the first grade from how they had been in kindergarten. Snack time was gone, and so was naptime. Instead of coloring and playing, we had to sit at our desks and do work from a difficult workbook. The work was not easy and it was hard to sit for so long.

Still, I liked school and enjoyed my classmates. Out on the PE field everything was fine. I was part of the crowd and had many friends. Everything was wonderful, but when I walked back into the classroom it all started going downhill again. I did not know what the problem was, but I knew something was wrong.

After a week or so, the teacher began teaching us the alphabet. She also taught us to write our names. I could not quite get the hang of it. Somehow my letters came out different from hers. First of all, it was easier to write from the right side of the page. Some letters turned themselves around and faced the wrong direction. I kept trying, but some invisible gremlin was messing up my work.

Next, we began studying phonics and learning to read. One day the teacher wrote the twenty-six symbols of the alphabet across the top of the board. Then she arranged some of the letters into three sentences of instructions and said, "do what these instructions tell you to do." I did exactly what the directions told me to do, nothing. I could not read the instructions. I did not understand them. I kept looking at them, thinking that by some magic I would be able to read those sentences, but I could not. It was clear that I was in big trouble.

That fear was confirmed when the teacher said, "Turn in your papers row by row."

I squirmed in my seat. The row on the far left of the room stood up and walked to the front to turn in their papers. The next row followed and walked single file to the teacher's desk. The teacher then called my row. I stood up. My mind raced as I tried to figure out what to do. My paper was blank. The consequences might be severe if I turned in a blank paper. I had a vision of the teacher yelling at me or worse telling the class that I could not read. I just could not risk that much embarrassment and humiliation. It was not a hard decision. I had to get out of there.

In fearful situations, we either fight or take flight. As a child, I thought that my only option was to run. As I stood up with my row, I saw that the previous row was heading back to their desks, passing by my desk. With the grace of a cat, I turned and stepped into that row. That row sat down and with my heart pounding in my chest, I kept walking until I reached the back of the room. I crouched down behind the dollhouse that served as a reading area, so the teacher could not see me. The dollhouse was about four feet tall, with the back cut out of it with books shoved in. I just crunched down behind it and no one knew I was there. I spent the next few minutes nervously folding my blank sheet of paper. I folded it, folded it again and refolded it until it was a tiny little ball, soaking wet from my sweaty palms. I was scared to death. School was not fun anymore.

I learned a valuable lesson that day, one that would stay with me throughout my early school years. I could hide from the teacher. In retrospect, I can see that those years would have been much different, and much less painful, if I had taken only one small step, which was the step to tell someone, "I can't read." When I tell this story to children, I always pause to tell them, "Do not take your problems on all by yourself. Tell your parents. Tell your teachers. Get help."

Over the years, I have learned that sharing a problem dilutes it. I have learned that the more people you ask to help you with a problem, the better chance you have of beating it. I should have told my parents. I should have told my teacher. But I was a child, with a child's mind and a child's fears. And I told no one.

The Bag of Tricks

That day in the first grade marked the beginning of what I now call my "bag of tricks." That "bag of tricks" soon expanded to include lying, cheating and memorizing. That is how I made it to the 5th grade without my teachers knowing, or so I thought, that I could not read.

It became second nature for me to invent stories to cover up the truth. Reading was more difficult, but that only meant I had to be more skilled. The reading group sat at a kidney shaped table. Each child would read a portion of the story so that everyone had a chance to read.

I was very anxious the first time I participated in this group. The first child was asked to read part of a typical See Spot Run story. Then the second and third children read and were corrected by the teacher. I was next and I could not read a word. However, I had listened carefully as the other children read. I picked up my book, wiped my wet palms, and tilted the book so the teacher could not see which page I was on. Then I recited the story verbatim, even making the corrections I had heard the teacher give the other children. The teacher announced that I read very well. In fact, she said I was an "advanced" reader. I knew I had just developed another tool for my "bag of tricks."

As a child, I had no idea how stressful it was for me to keep the secret that I could not read. But I did know I was deceiving my teacher, and more importantly, I was deceiving my family that loved and supported me. It was not easy to like myself.

Each morning my mother got me up for school and each morning I did not want to go. I felt nauseated and physically sick each and every day. Half way through the first grade, I broke out in raised purple whelps all down my legs, my legs and feet were swollen. After weeks of doctors and tests I was diagnosed with a rare blood disease that without bed rest could permanently damage my kidneys. I was out of school for six weeks, just short of the time it took to qualify for a home bound teacher. I was happy and relieved that I did not have to go to school while they tried to diagnose and treat me. I fervently wished that it would be a long time before a cure was found. No such luck. Within six weeks, I was back in school. No doubt this illness was the result of stress of a child not being able to cope.

After first grade, the teacher gave my mom a list of about 200 words to go over with me during the summer "so I would not forget them." There was nothing to forget. The only words I recognized on the list was "A" and "I." As a seven- year-old I had faked my way through first grade. It was a milestone, and the process would continue for several years. No one could say I was dumb. It takes a smart kid to dupe adults.

This was the beginning of my tutoring years. Mom immediately found a tutor three mornings a week for the summer. At the end of summer I could recognize more words but still could barely read a three-word sentence. The tutor was a teacher from another county. At the end of the summer she told my mother that she had used every method she knew in addition to asking for advice from other teacher friends. She said she knew I was smart but could not find a way to teach me to read.

Mom's Determination

My first experience with an IQ test came in the 2nd grade. One day, my teacher walked up to me and said, "Rob, we need to give you a test."

"Okay," I said.

Then she said the frightful words."Come with me. You will take the test alone in another room."

In each class, I had my "cheat group" and a "test taking position." I always sat forward at my desk, and my friends agreed to leave their papers uncovered so I could copy from them. I passed the spelling and math tests this way. My teacher would ask me if I was cheating and, with practiced innocence, I would say, "No, ma'am."

Leaving the room to take a test terrified me. This took me out of my cheat group. I lagged behind as we walked down the hall to the media center. My heart raced and I began to sweat. We sat down, the teacher and I. Even then, I recognized that it does not matter how smart you are or how many tricks you have, you are not going to fool a teacher one-on-one.

I grabbed the pencil, and had trouble holding it because of my slippery hands. As I took the test, I knew I was not doing well. My teacher did not give me my score, but the next day my mom was called in for a conference. The teacher told her that I had scored an 84 on the IQ test. (A reporter writing my story for a local newspaper, later in my life, described my IQ as being a small step above Forrest Gump.)

The teacher told Mom, "We are worried about Rob. We do not think he has the intelligence to make it in regular classes. Maybe he should be put in a self contained LD class.

The explosion that followed was my mother telling the teacher off. My mom was livid. Red with anger and tears streaming down her face, she said, "My son is smart at home but failing at school. There must be something wrong with the way you teach him. Rob will not be placed in a special SLD program. Nor will he be singled out as a mentally handicapped child."

The teacher was surprised at this response, and I continued as a regular student in her class.

My mother was not an expert in learning disabilities. At that time we did not even know I had a learning disability.

But it was about this time that my father's mother told my mom that my dad's teacher in 3rd grade had told her that he was "mirror eyed" and there was nothing they could do for that. This was mom's first clue towards the learning disability of dyslexia. Mom became determined, and she was focused. Her focus that day and throughout my entire educational career was: What needs to happen for my child to learn in school today?

On that particular day, it meant staying in school. On other days, it meant other things. Mom's persistence took many forms over the years, but it always answered the question: What needs to happen for my child to learn in school today?

Somewhere my parents heard about an ophthalmologist who claimed to be able to teach a child like me to read through exercises and reinforced phonics. I was taken two afternoons a week for the remainder of the school year to a nearby town to work with this doctor. In addition, the reading specialist in my school tutored me one hour a day. The results were minimal at best.

In 3rd grade, Mom got me into a program at the county office one afternoon a week, after school. This was a one-on-one with a county reading specialist. After a year of this tutoring, the results remained minimal.

I Can't Write What I Know

The commitment to my getting what I needed in order to learn showed up again a few years later, and provided a breakthrough; it was our first clue as to what to do about my trouble in school.

Every evening after dinner, Mom and I would trek up the stairs to my room to begin our nightly routine of studying the next day's assignments or for a test. Sometimes another family member would help, but usually it was Mom.

On one particularly cold winter night when I was in 5th grade, Mom and I plumped up the pillows on my bed, made our comfortable nest, and talked about the day's activities. This preliminary talk was our way of gearing up to tackle my schoolwork. Mom listened attentively and, no matter what I told her, was accepting and non-judgmental. We were relaxed and I felt safe enough to be myself. Even as I grew up, Mom and I often met in the kitchen late at night to talk into the wee hours of the morning. I would confide in her, as do many of her friends, because she is a great listener and never criticizes.

I never dreaded this study time, even though the lessons were difficult for me. Mom and I shared the same vision of my being successful in school. We were a team. If I had to study for a test, Mom asked what the teacher wanted and expected. After I told her, she read the textbook, the syllabus, or other information to me. She read and read and read until her voice became hoarse. Sometimes it was completely gone by the time we finished studying.

After reading the lessons, we discussed the contents and summarized the major points. The final step came when Mom asked me questions as if I was taking the test. After several hours of studying that night, she said, "You've got it. You know the material backwards and forwards."

The next day I went to school and confidently entered my history class, expecting to ace the test. Mom had said I knew the material. The teacher handed out a paper with twenty questions requiring essay answers. I tackled the test and did the best I could, but I could not finish the answers in the allotted time.

I was not eager to go to this class the following day because the teacher was giving back our test and I suspected that I had not made a good grade. It was worse than I thought. Not only had I not done well, I had failed the test.

When I arrived home from school that afternoon, Mom could tell that something was wrong from my hang-dog expression. I showed her the test and she was extremely puzzled.

"You only have answers to two of the questions and those are incomplete," she said. "Rob, I know you know this material, but this test does not reflect that. What happened?" I thought about it and finally blurted out the essence of the problem.

"Mom, I can't write what I know."

Discovering A Learning Style

It was just that simple. I could not write what I knew. That is a learning style. If you can not write what you know, you have to find another way to be understood. For me, that way was oral testing. If the teacher asked me the questions verbally, and I was allowed to speak the answer, I could say what I knew. I just could not write what I knew.

The day after I got my failing grade on that history test, Mom went to school with me and said to the teacher, "If you read the questions to Rob and he gives you satisfactory answers, will you give him credit for knowing the answers?"

The teacher said, "Yes."

She read the questions to me and I told her every answer. I got 100% on that test. My teacher said, "Rob does know this stuff!" I lit up like a light. That is exactly what I needed to hear. My self-esteem skyrocketed. It was very important to me that my teacher thought I was smart. It changed everything.

And something else changed, too. We had set a precedent. I had no idea until much later how important that would be, but we had set the precedent of oral testing. From that point on, they had to let me take tests orally. For someone who cannot write what he knows, oral testing makes all the difference, because I had a way to succeed.

This was the first of many discoveries we made, and many ups and downs along the way. Mom had arrangements with my teacher for me to take my next test in a separate classroom. She and I studied the night before and I knew the material. But the next day, I was given the test with the rest of the class. Everyone finished the test except me, and the class was dismissed into free time. Everybody was running around, and making all the noise that 5th graders make during free time. I could no longer think, so I turned my paper in.

The next day I brought home an "F" and mom asked why I had failed. I told her what had happened and she was furious. She took me to school the next morning and asked the teacher why I had not been tested the way they had agreed. The teacher said she had too many students to test me alone.

Mom just stood there and looked at her for a minute. Then she said, "Well, I am withdrawing him from school."

"You can not do that," the teacher said. "It is against the law."

"Watch me!" Mom said, simply. With that she handed the teacher my books, took my arm and walked away.

Mom and I knew something the teacher did not. We had already moved to Rockdale County and I was only staying there until the semester ended in two more weeks.

Learning that I am Smart

Before moving Mom had already talked to the principal and reading specialist at the new school. I expected more of the same after we moved, but my mother promised me that this school would be different. I did not believe her. The morning I was supposed to start at the new school, Mom walked into my room and asked, "Are you ready to go to school?"

"No," I said. She wanted to know why I did not want to go.

"Because I am terrible in school. I don't like it."

Mom said again that this school was going to be different. I still did not believe her.

"How?" I asked.

"The teachers are going to listen to you. They are not going to make you feel dumb. They are going to answer your questions and they are going to care."

That was hard for me to believe. It was a tall order. But Mom had always been straight with me, so I decided to give this new school a chance. It was one of those "character building moments."

I walked awkwardly into the 5th grade class. I was the new kid, coming in at the middle of the year, and this was my first day. The teacher greeted me pleasantly and then said, "I need to give you a test."

With a heavy heart, I answered, "Let me guess, the placement test?"

"Yes," she said.

I gathered my courage and said, "Well, I don't want to take it."

"Why?" She asked, surprised. I told her that I had done "bad" on it before.

"We are going to do it differently," she said with a smile.

"Differently?" I asked.

"Yes, we are going to give you blocks and puzzles to work with and we will time you. Then we will sit down and talk to you and see what you can do." Feeling encouraged but still a little skeptical, I followed her to the media center. The tester clicked the clock and I arranged the blocks as instructed. When we finished, we had a nice long conversation.

The next day, the teacher called my parents in for a conference. All I could think was, "Oh no. Here we go again. They are going to make Mom mad and we are going to be moving again." I was wrong.

"Rob, do you know that you are really smart?" the teacher asked.

"Really?" I replied with shock.

She repeated the magical sentence. "You are very smart."

Practically speechless, I again uttered, "Really?"

She assured me that it was true. My mother and father smiled the biggest smile I had ever seen on their faces. I thought, "It must be true."

For the rest of my 5th grade year, I was taken out of my English class. Instead, I went to the media center to be tutored in reading. At the end of the year, I expressed my concern to the reading specialist about what was going to happen when I entered 6th grade in middle school. Because of my anxiety, she wrote a wonderful letter to Edwards Middle School that paved the way for their understand of my disability.

The Phil Donahue Show

When I was in school, we did not know as much about dyslexia as we do today. My mom was always on the lookout for information about what might be wrong with me, but we did not know quite what we were looking for so we learned slowly and somewhat haphazardly. One day my grandmother was watching the Phil Donahue Show, and a Dr. Harold Levinson came on with Bruce Jenner, the Olympic athlete, to talk about dyslexia. She said to herself, "My goodness, that Bruce Jenner sounds so much like Rob."

She told my mother, who went to the school and said, "I want Rob tested for dyslexia." The school agreed to the test, but told her there was a three year waiting list. If they had said this to anyone else, they might have given up. But Mom called the Phil Donahue Show and said; "I need a transcript of the show with Harold Levinson as a guest."

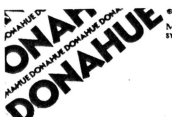

MULTIMEDIA PROGRAM PRODUCTIONS
SYNDICATION SERVICES P.O. BOX 2111 CINCINNATI, OHIO 45201

DONAHUE TRANSCRIPT #08171

APPEARANCES: Mr. Phil Donahue
Harold Levinson
(Ph.D.)
Mr. Bruce Jenner
Christian Sachs
Mrs. Rita Sachs
Rosalind Schwartz
(Mrs.)
Bari-Joy Schwartz
Mrs. Roberta Rebhun
Laura Levinson

)

Phil Donahue: Doctor Harold Levinson has come up with a fascinating and much discussed, and has attracked the attention of the porfessional community with his thesis that children or anybody with dyslexia has an inner ear dysfunction. What is fascinating about this, ah--what's important about this is a whole lot of people have dyslexia. We can only guess or wonder how many young children are in school being accused of laziness, whose parents have had it suggested that they are LD, learning disabilities. We have letters now to identify all kinds of things that we don't really understand. Not to mention children who have been--it has been suggested have emotional problems, maybe even brain damage. Now, many, many young people are carrying these burdens of failure through the formative years, and are emotionally crippled by the time they get to be eighteen, twenty-two years old. They have come to believe that they are no good, when the fact is that they may have a physical difficulty that has largely gone undiscovered, lo these many years. How am I doing so far, Doctor?

Harold Levinson: Wonderful!

Phil Donahue: Yeah?

Harold Levinson: I hope I can follow.

Phil Donahue: Okay.

Audience: (Loud laughter)

Phil Donahue: First of all, give me some of the--dyslexics can't read or have difficulty reading?

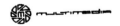

28

Sure enough, they sent her the transcript. She read it and called Dr. Levinson, who was a pioneer in the field of dyslexia. She said, "I hear you test for dyslexia." He said he did and Mom said, "I need you to prove my son has dyslexia."

What gave her that kind of courage? She knew then what we know now: if her child did not make it in education, he was not going to make it at all. Nothing was out of bounds for my mother, because she was going to make sure that her child made it. Again, it boiled down to, "What needs to happen for my child to learn in school today?" That day, we needed for Dr. Levinson to prove that I was dyslexic so she could start getting me what we would later call accommodations." Mom was not interested in Dr. Levinson's theories, but she did know I could get more services from the school system if I had a diagnosis of dyslexia. Mom had found out that I could get all of my books on tape from The Library for the Blind but at that time she was told that she had to have a diagnosis from an M.D. in order for me to qualify.

My parents scraped together the money for my dad, my brother and me to fly to New York for the appointment with Dr. Levinson. We did not have a lot of money at that time, but I now realize that my parents probably would have sold our house if that is what it took to get us to New York.

Dr. Levinson believed that dyslexia was caused by an inner ear problem. He ran water in my ears and I counted pink elephants flying across the wall in front of me. He said I had "Cerebeller-Vestibular Dysfunction." This was a diagnosis supporting dyslexia from a medical doctor. (We never filled Dr. Levinson's prescription for antihistamines.)

For the Children

HAROLD N. LEVINSON, M.D., P.C.
FRESH MEADOWS PROFESSIONAL BUILDING
61-34 188TH STREET
FRESH MEADOWS, NEW YORK 11365
—
TELEPHONE 454-4848

Dear Correspondent:

As a result of the influx of individuals interested and inquiring about Dr. Levinson's methods of diagnosing and treating dyslexic individuals, this form letter was expediently drafted.

The diagnostic procedure takes approximately 2½ hours and is completed in one visit. It includes all neurological, ocular, "inner ear" and psycho-educational testing to make an adequate diagnosis. This diagnosis can be made and explained in almost 100% of the cases seen.

In addition, a treatment plan is determined on the basis of the test findings. Thus far, 75% of individuals will have a favorable therapeutic response to various combinations of medications and 25% will not. The favorable response will vary from mild to dramatic, and is thus far not predictable.

The total fee for this diagnostic-treatment evaluation, performed by Dr. Levinson or his associate, is $500. This fee _must_ be paid at the time of the examination. All testing is medical, and may be reimbursable according to the manner in which your particular insurance policy covers you for other out-of-hospital medical services.

At the present time, Dr. Levinson and his associate are the only physicians performing the above described diagnosis and treatment.

I hope this letter clearly explains Dr. Levinson's office procedure. Should you have any questions, please write or phone.

Sincerely yours,

Carolyn

Carolyn
Secretary to Dr. Levinson

P.S. To insure proper testing, all individuals with appointments should:
1. be medication free for 24 hours - if possible,
2. eat lightly prior to testing, and
3. if you have a tendency to accumulate wax, have your physician check and clean your ears.

30

Redefining Success in School and Success in Life

NAME _Robert Langston_   AGE _____ DATE _5/9/83_

MEDICAL INSTRUCTIONS

Medication is to be taken as follows:

(1a) _Meclizine   25   ¼_ Tablets/ _1_ X DAY

AM ✓
NOON
3-4 PM ✓

Increase the dosage slowly (three day intervals) to:
_¼_ OR _1_ Tablets/ _1_ X Day, if possible within a two-week period providing no side effects occur.*

(1b) After _1_ weeks, ADD (1b) _Persantine 100mg (¼-½-1) 2x1_

(1c) After _3_ weeks, ADD (1c) _[handwritten] 1200mg 1x1 day_

(2) After _4_ weeks, ADD (2) _Cylert (¼-½-1) 1x/daily_

(3) After _____ weeks, ADD (3) _____

*<u>Possible Side Effects</u> are: Tiredness, irritability, sleepiness, insomnia, etc. If any of these symptoms occur, reduce medication to the previous dose, or to one-half of the original starting dose. If the symptoms persist, stop the medication and move on to the next medication.

If you have any questions regarding medication, call Monday through Friday during office hours. (New York Time) 8:30 AM to 5:00 PM. If I am busy at the time of your call, my nurse will schedule you for a specific call back time.

Send us the progress report given you at our office _8_ weeks after your visit.

Re-visit: Patient should be reexamined in _12_ months ON _✓_/OFF _____ medication. There is an additional fee for the second visit.

All medications may lead to reversible side effects - especially if the dose is too high. These side effects can be avoided by means of lowering the dose. <u>No dose is too low</u> if the patient is sensitive to the medication. A positive response may be obtained despite a low dose. Medication should be taken with food. If lowering the dose does not help, eliminate the medication and move on to the next medication prescribed.

Any patient on Cylert or Pemoline should have a SMAC (Liver Profile) blood test performed locally every three months. The results should be sent to your local physician and myself.

IMPORTANT: After 8 weeks of favorable response- medication is to be discontinued on weekends, holidays and vacations (Summers), or lowered on those occasions only. (Regular routine during weekdays.) If attending school during vacations & summers, or, if work is done weekends, medications may be taken in regular or half doses.
When resuming medication after long intervals, resume at half the dosage for three days and then you may return to maximum at time you discontinued.

Please feel free to contact us should you have any questions.

Thank you.

HAROLD N. LEVINSON, M.D. P.C.

For the Children

National Library Service for the
Blind and Physically Handicapped
The Library of Congress   LIBRARY FOR THE BLIND AND PHYSICALLY HANDICAPPED
Washington, D.C. 20542   THE NEW YORK PUBLIC LIBRARY
202-882-5500   166 AVENUE OF THE AMERICAS
NEW YORK, N.Y. 10013

Application for Free Library Service—Individuals

Notice: Records relating to recipients of Library of Congress reading material are confidential except for those portions defined by local law as public information. To find out the extent to which the information provided on this application form may be released to other individuals, institutions, or agencies, consult the agency to which you are submitting this application. If you do not know that address, send the completed application to the Library of Congress. It will be forwarded to the appropriate agency.

Please print or type:
Name _____ Telephone _____
  (last)   (first)   (initial)

Address _____
  (street)   (city)   (state)   (zip code)

Date of birth _____ Sex _____

By law, preference in the lending of books and equipment is given to veterans. Please check here if you have been honorably discharged from the armed forces of the United States. □

Indicate the disability preventing you from reading standard printed material. See definitions under eligibility criteria on page 4.

□ blindness   □ visual handicap   □ physical handicap   ☑ reading disability

In addition to any of the above conditions, do you also have a hearing impairment? If yes, indicate the degree of hearing loss:
  □ moderate(some difficulty hearing and understanding speech)
  □ profound(cannot hear or understand speech)

over   73—101(rev 9/78)

Reading Preferences

To help your library begin serving you, information is needed about your general reading interests. Check the types of books you prefer, or write your reading interests in the space provided:

- ☐ current novels
- ☐ historical novels
- ☐ family stories
- ☐ mysteries
- ☐ westerns

- ☐ short stories
- ☐ poetry
- ☐ Bible and religion
- ☐ biography
- ☐ history and travel

- ☐ science and nature
- ☐ current affairs
- ☐ books in foreign languages (specify the language)

_____

Other reading interests_____

_____

☐ Send only books I request, indicated above.   ☐ Select books for me in the subject areas

To Be Completed by Certifying Authority

I certify that the applicant named is unable to read or use standard printed material for the reason(s) indicated on page one of this form.

_____
(signature)

_____
(title and occupation)

HAROLD N. LEVINSON, M.D., P.C.
600 NORTHERN BLVD.
GREAT NECK, N.Y. 11021
516-482-2888

_____
address

_____
(city)   (state)   (zip code)

_____
over   (date)

I am a great believer in getting tested by people outside the school system. We have to change the system, but sometimes the system does not like to change from within. Sometimes it takes outside influences. My mother knew that in order for people to give me what I needed, they had to hear that I was dyslexic. She also knew that if she waited three years until the school was ready to give me the test, it might be too late. She fixed it so that people were told what they needed to hear in order for me to become a lifetime learner.

Today a child does not have to have a M.D. diagnosis in order to get accommodations, but at that time you did.

Pieces of the Puzzle

Fear and learning do not go together. When you are frightened, you just cannot learn, but my mother became a master at taking fear out of the classroom.

In school one day the teacher was going up and down the rows calling on each student in turn to read aloud a paragraph of a story. I always tried to figure out which paragraph we would be on by the time it got to me. That day I was practicing the paragraph I knew would be mine, struggling to decipher the words and letters. Suddenly the teacher skipped a student. She went out of order! She skipped Johnny! Now I would not get the paragraph I had been practicing! I panicked, because nobody really understood that I could not read well and I did not want my friends to know.

Sure enough, the teacher called on me. I had not had a chance to practice the new paragraph and I did a poor job of reading it. I went home that afternoon feeling very low and mom asked me what had happened.

"Well, Mom, the teacher called on me to read," I said.

The next day mom went to the school and got the teacher to agree not to call on me to read aloud in class. Being asked to read aloud in front of my classmates was terrifying to me. Mom understood that removing one fear made it easier for me to learn. Mom then told me that if I was called on to read again that I could politely say, "I do not want to read aloud."

I went back to class the next day and again we started reading up and down the rows. I was listening to this wonderful story and instead of sweating bullets for fear of being called on, I was actually understanding what was being read and loving it. I retain 85% of what I know from listening. That is my learning style. When it was my turn, I just said, "Remember me? I'd rather not read aloud in class." The teacher smiled and never called on me again.

That took all the fear out of that class for me and I was free to learn. My teacher understood that and held onto that piece of the puzzle for me; I did not have to read aloud in class. My mother was already holding a lot of the pieces of my puzzle; separate classrooms, oral testing, etc. She would tell me, "Rob, this is how you learn. Do it this way when you go to college."

There was never any thought that I would not go to college. I remember back when I was in high school, and some of my friends were talking about what they were going to do after graduation. It did not include college. I asked my mom, "Can they do that? Could you just not go to college?"

A Special Student

In middle school, they told me, "You are a special person and we are going to give you your own classroom for one period a day. And we are going to give you your own personal teacher."

That sounded great until the teacher escorted me down the hall to my "special" classroom. Puzzled, I looked into the 4" x 6" room and saw a dirty sink on the wall. The odor of cleaning supplies permeated the air. Mops and brooms were stacked in the corner. It was the janitor's closet. I began to doubt the school's motives. Did they really believe I was smart? Did they really have my best interests at heart? Being new to this school and having been burned in the past, I had no confidence that they were treating me fairly.

They decided to clean up the room. They took the sink off the wall and brought in two desks and chairs. This was to be my classroom for special help for one period each day. I would go there and sit with a teacher and she would ask me questions. I answered her orally and if I knew the material I passed even if I could not write it down.

But I had another problem. What if my friend's saw me walk into a janitor's closet for class? What would they think? My social future at this school might be jeopardized if my friends discovered my disability. I decided it was time for me to start testing the waters as my own advocate and assuming responsibility for my own success, so I went to my regular classroom teacher with a request.

"Ah, you know, I am a special person," I began.

"Yes?" She said, looking a little suspicious.

I worked up my courage and continued. "Because I am special, I have this special classroom."

Again she said, "Yes?" I could tell she wondered what I was up to.

With bravado I did not feel, I said, "I also need a special time to go to my special class." She looked doubtful.

"What do you mean?"

"I need to go to class five minutes late," I said. She let me know in no uncertain terms that this was impossible.

"Nobody, not even special people, go to class five minutes late," she said. But she was looking past my words to my anxiety and kindly asked me what the real problem was.

"I am embarrassed for my friends to see me going into the janitor's closet to learn," I confessed. It was a huge risk. I had not told the truth in the past and had not had success with it up to that point. But amazingly, the truth worked. She gave me permission to go to class five minutes after all the other students were settled into their classes. I had dodged another social bullet. Each day when the bell rang I looked very busy as I waved good-bye to my friends. As soon as the hall cleared, I headed down to my closet for my hour of one-on-one attention from the teacher.

I had many friends at school and was involved in many activities, but I was still cheating and hiding. I was cheating myself from having open, honest relationships with my friends. I was hiding the real me, the me with learning disabilities. I soon learned that life has a way of calling your bluff and unmasking the truth.

My Moment of Truth

My day of reckoning came during my first year in middle school. Every day after school, my friends and I would go down to the local gas station to play video games. I loved video games and was very good at them. I was the video game wizard in our group.

One Wednesday afternoon after school, my friends and I rode our bikes the two miles to the gas station where we played video games. As we stood around talking, inhaling cokes and peanuts, a deliveryman came in pushing a large hand truck with a new video game on it. We could hardly contain our excitement as we gathered around to watch him plug in the new Donkey Kong game.

My friends said, "Rob, you go first. You're best at the video games." So I stepped up to the game, fascinated as I watched the brilliant display of flashing lights. I grabbed the joysticks and inserted my quarters. The screen came up.

All of a sudden, I thought I was going to faint. Nausea swept through my body and panic set in. I stared at the screen. It might as well have been written in Swahili. I could not read the instructions.

My friends waited expectantly while my mind raced. What should I do? I could not run away. I was going to have to stay and fight. I turned to my best friend and said, "Brian, I have this thing, a learning disability. It is called dyslexia. What it means is I don't read too well. Do you think you can help me out and read these instructions to me?"

You could have heard a pin drop. Brian looked at me, and then looked down at his feet. I thought, 'What have you done? They are not going to be your friends anymore. They are going to find out you are different and they will not like someone with a learning disability. They will laugh at you.'

After what seemed an eternity, Brian looked me squarely in the eye and said, "You know, I think I have heard of that. Yeah, sure, I'll read the instructions. You can still go first." My relief was so great that I could have hugged him.

That was a monumental day for me, because I realized that my friends did not care if I learned differently. All they cared about was that I was Rob. They wanted to be with the "real" Rob. It was another life-changing, "character building moment." Suddenly, I did not have to hide and cheat anymore. My friends knew the real me and accepted me just the way I was.

When I tell my story to young people, I usually preface it by saying, "I am going to tell you how not to do it," and then I go on to tell about the lying, cheating, and hiding. But when I come to this part of the story, I say, "This is how you do it. You tell the truth. You let people support you."

Some time later I was riding the bus with Brian, and for some reason, I wrote down his name. I wrote it: "Brain." Brian glanced over, saw his name misspelled and commented, "I wish I was a "brain." It was a very kind thing to say and another confirmation that my friends accepted me even with my disability.

With both my teachers and my friends helping me, I began to see that the more people you have helping you solve your problems, the better off you are. It is vitally important for students with learning disabilities to tell their parents and teachers so they can help. We all have problems in life, and we all learn differently. We all struggle in different areas, and we can all help one another.

The Key is Self-esteem

My mother knew intuitively that there were two keys to my success:

Maintain Rob's self-esteem. Self-esteem is the most important issue in everyone's life. I went for a large portion of my life without it and I have seen that many other people go without it as well. You simply cannot survive in life without your self-esteem. That was my mother's attitude:

"Keep my child's self-esteem intact." It is the best advice I can give any parent of a learning disabled child.

Get him what he needs to learn in class today. Today, the law requires that we provide "free, appropriate public education" to everyone, but there is a lot of bureaucracy and red tape involved. That red tape is killing students. My mother was a master at cutting through red tape, and she did it by focusing on this principle.

Mom did not let anyone or anything get in the way of the key to success. She kept her focus on my self-esteem and on today's lessons, and that is what made her so powerful. She taught me the same focus and that attitude made me a lifelong learner.

CHAPTER 3

Learning About Myself: High School

At the beginning of high school, Mom announced to my teachers, "Rob has to go to college." As I said, she had always had an unequivocal belief that I was going to college and I had grown up thinking that everyone went to college.

I had been left on the waiting list for county testing, even though Dr. Levinson had privately diagnosed me. It was 9th grade when my number came up. I was taken to the county office for one-on-one testing by a county specialist. She started out testing me with reading but went back to the blocks and puzzles. A few weeks later my parents and I were called back for the results. The specialist confirmed a learning disability. She said that my reading skills were so low that she was unable to give me an exact score but that my IQ was in the high superior range. The next step was a meeting with all my teachers, the school reading specialist, counselor, my parents and a county representative to decide what to do for me. They went around the table giving each teacher a chance to give his or her analysis on what they had seen in their class. The two teachers who had me for classes that required no reading were shocked when they got the notice for a LD meeting on me. Neither had seen any signs of a problem in their classes. At the end, the school LD teacher stood and said that she had gone over all the test results and her recommendation was to have me in her LD class one or two periods a day and she was sure she could teach me to read on my grade level. My mother had sat quietly with tears in her eyes listening to yet another conference listing her child's weaknesses. The LD teacher had all her recommendations written down and handed them to my parents to sign so that she could get started. Mom pushed the paper away and said she would not sign. There was silence. The teacher then pushed the paper toward Dad who picked up a pen. Mom took the pen and stood up indicating the meeting was over. Finally the LD teacher asked Mom what she wanted done. Mom says now that she does not know where it came from, but at that moment she was convinced that, "after all the things that had been done through the years for my reading skills, actually teaching me to read had ceased to be an option." She said, "I want to bypass his eyes altogether and have him taught orally."

The LD teacher thought a minute and said, "I can not do that."

Mom said, "Then I will have to find another way." Then, she and Dad walked out.

A few days later the LD teacher called mom and said she was willing to try what she wanted. It was decided that I would go to the LD classroom the last period of the day. All my teachers would send their tests to her to be given to me orally and she would also help me with homework if I needed help. My mother believes that this was the turning point of my academic career.

For years teachers had been trying to teach me to read with no success. I had been going to a regular school for six hours a day and to a special school for learning to read two hours a day. I had studied phonics daily during my English class period and worked with a tutor every summer since 1st grade. Mom had investigated many "cure-all" treatments and tried anything that sounded like it might work, but still I could not read.

Each teacher thought that if they just taught me a little longer and/or a little harder, I would master reading. But it never happened. They were beating a dead horse, trying to make something work by doing something that obviously did not work. In essence, the teachers had continued to focus on my weakness rather than on my strengths.

Part of Mom's decision that I would no longer be taught to read was that with each failure, my self-esteem took a blow. In light of these facts, her decision was not frivolous. It was simply based on supporting my self-esteem while finding a way for me to learn. She intuitively knew that self-esteem was the most important element of success and she always protected me when the standard operating procedures of the educational system might have destroyed it.

At that time, the school system did not understand that we all have different learning styles. Teachers simply taught by reading the same way teachers had always taught. The assumption was that all children learn the same way. However, recent studies have proven that this assumption is not correct.

There are multiple ways of learning, multiple doors leading into the brain. For some, the door may be through the eyes. For others, it may be through the ears. For others, the door is through moving, touching and experiencing. Smell and taste can also be a part of learning. My mother was determined that my learning style, which is primarily auditory that is learning by listening, would be honored.

High school brought a whole new set of lessons and understandings. But first, we had to revisit some old ground.

Oral Testing, Again

Battles that had been won in elementary and middle school sometimes had to be fought again in high school. One of them was oral testing.

Dr. Roger Newton's Science class was typical of my high school experiences. I was making 20's and 30's on tests and, consequently, failing the class. When Mom discovered this, she called to set up a conference for my dad and her with Dr. Newton to discuss how I could improve my grades.

Mom and Dad met with Dr. Newton one afternoon and while Dr. Newton was going over my test scores, my mother was looking over his shoulder at his test scores book. She saw that over one third of the class was failing. She immediately brought it to his attention that the problem must be his inability to relate to the students on their level. He was very defensive and said that his other classes were doing passing work. After everyone calmed down he agreed to meet me before school to go over each chapter and give me an oral test. After one quarter of doing this, Dr. Newton wrote my parents a letter that said, "Rob's test grades this quarter have been 84%, 84% and 92%, a fantastic improvement. Morning sessions have worked so well. I think it has been a massive improvement with a minimum of time expense. I will continue to give him his tests orally, which has been the major difference in his progress."

11-15-82

Mr & Mrs. Langstm,

Rob's test grades this quarter have been 84, 84, 92 — a fantastic improvement! I am pleased with his progress. I have found that Rob "catches on" quickly to the science concepts/problems, but that he often has <u>major</u> misconceptions that are <u>easy</u> to correct. That's why our morning sessions have worked so well. I think it has been a massive improvement with a minimum of time expense. I would like to continue these sessions on <u>Thursday</u> each week (whenever he gets to school). [On difficult chapters, perhaps we may need an extra day or so.] I will continue to give his tests orally — that has been the other major difference in his progress. TEST 4 will be <u>Tuesday</u> 11/23 (due to the holidays).

Sincerely, Roger Newton

45

Looking at the teachers that stand out at times of struggle in my educational career, I began to realize there were some teachers mom and I struggled with and many teachers that we didn't struggle with at all. Since this book is about the struggles facing education today, the teachers that stood out most were the ones that had either a little extra patience, a little more persistence, or both. As with Dr. Newton, sometimes questioning motives can force results.

The question posed to Dr. Newton from Mom gave him the incentive to prove or disprove the facts. Lucky for me, Dr. Newton was a science teacher and this approach appealed to him. The situation was to prove or disprove that I could get better grades with some minor accommodations. The difference between the teachers I struggled with, and never saw again (because I was pulled from their class) and the teachers I struggled with, but ultimately found success, was due to their willingness to try something different. Mom's ability to fight was irrelevant if the teacher wasn't willing to cooperate. The trademark of the teachers profiled here is that they were willing to try something new.

Dr. Newton is more than just another accommodations success story. He is the epitome of accommodations success because his positive contribution to me did not stop at just his grade book. When I speak to teachers I pose the question, "Can one teacher make a difference?". And I think we all know what the answer is...YES! But the thing I kept hearing from teachers over my first decade of speaking was, I don't mind doing it in my classroom, but will it make a difference down the road? And my answer is Dr. Newton. He not only made the necessary accommodations in his class, but he documented it with the letter reprinted in this book.

To this day I have kept all my school records. When I opened my folder, it was the first thing that fell out. I had to ask myself how this letter had survived two years of high school and seven years of college in my permanent record. I called my mom and said, "You won't believe what has been saved in my records!". When I told her about the letter, she said "I know." I asked how she knew, and she said, "because I requested it be put there." She somehow knew that the hand-written letter would set the precedent for me to be able to take my SAT test without time restrictions, and in a separate class, with a reader. The letter also served me in college because it allowed me to take the Regents test the same way. Is setting the precedent that enabled me to level the playing field on standardized testing enough to land Dr. Newton as "one of the most important people in my educational career?" Answer, "You Bet!" Can one teacher make a lasting difference in a student's life? Answer, "You Bet!"

Not only was the oral testing precedent established but my self-esteem was preserved. It was very important to me that my teachers knew and acknowledged that I was intelligent. Before a teacher discovered that I was smart, I could tell from their words and tone that they did not think I measured up. That was terrible for my self-esteem. I sometimes felt like I was dying inside.

Even when precedents were established and teachers were aware of my learning style; not all teachers were willing to help me. But "No," was never the final answer because my mother did not accept it. Mom would dig in her heels, set her jaw and go on a search to find teachers who were cooperative. Mom says she was "stubborn." I say she was inspired!

At the beginning of each semester Mom and I would meet with the counselor and set up my schedule including choosing the teachers who best suited my needs. Then Mom would meet with new teachers and tell them about my learning style. When I reached college, I used my mom's example and conducted a relentless search to find professors who would work with me so that I could learn.

The Three-Step Formula

I believe that three elements must be in place before learning disabled students can succeed in school: communications, learning styles and precedents. By high school, Mom and I had established all three.

I had started communicating with my mom the minute I said to her in elementary school, "Mom, I can't write what I know." From that point on, we had an open and honest communication. I told her what my problems were, and she did her best to help me fix them. I no longer hid things from her or tried to cheat or lie to her.

We had also gotten some good information about my learning style. I was primarily an auditory learner. I received 85% of everything I learned from listening, so that was the best way for me to learn.

And we had begun to set precedents. We had in place: separate classrooms, oral testing and other accommodations like not having to read aloud in class.

It was a good beginning. We would keep working on all three.

New Challenges

Just knowing about my learning styles was not always enough. One of my teachers would not agree to oral testing, but she did agree to give me as much time as I needed to take the test. I had studied hard, memorizing every possible answer and even memorizing the spelling of all the words. But when the bell rang at the end of the period, I had finished only five of twenty questions.

My classmates stood up and filed out of the room. One of my friends called out, "Come on Rob. You'll miss the break. And weren't you going to ask Elizabeth to the prom?"

I was left sitting in the classroom by myself. I could not believe that it had taken me one hour to write five answers. I tried to write faster, but that just made me more anxious. The bell rang again and the next class filed in. The student who was supposed to be sitting in my seat during this period just sat on the floor, and I started to feel embarrassed.

I asked the teacher what I should do and she replied, "I agreed to give you extended time instead of oral testing, so stay where you are and continue."

The student whose seat I was sitting in was beginning to get miffed that he had been displaced. Others in the class were staring at me, wondering what I was doing in their class. The teacher began teaching the new class and I was further distracted. My discomfort was so great that I panicked and turned in the test incomplete. With great relief, I walked out the door.

Was my having to take the test in that way a major obstacle to my learning? You bet it was. It affected not only my learning, but also my relationships with my friends. My social standing may seem incidental to education, but it was not incidental to me as a learning disabled student, whose self-esteem had taken a beating for many years. In fact, at that time of my life, my social standing was a top priority. What was the answer? I needed a separate classroom for testing. When I got that accommodation, I could learn and succeed.

Walking on Fire

High school is a time when we all start growing up emotionally. I was no exception.

When I was sixteen, my father took me to Anthony Robbins' Firewalk Seminar. I learned that walking on fire is a metaphor for taking charge of your life by changing your belief system.[2] Tony taught us that even seemingly impossible tasks like walking on hot coals could be accomplished by internalizing a new belief. In this case, it was "I can successfully walk on hot coals."

Over the weekend seminar, Mr. Robbins drilled this idea into our subconscious minds until we actually believed it. Then he modeled that it could be done. And we demonstrated that we had learned our lessons well by doing the impossible, walking on hot coals without being burned. I walked on fire! The seemingly impossible was now possible. More importantly, I gained the knowledge, experience and courage to tackle tasks that had seemed beyond me only months earlier.

In addition to the Firewalk Seminar, my mother took me to a psychologist/hypnotherapist, supposedly to help me learn better, but really to help me deal with my anger and frustration.

Dr. Ron: A Whole New World

I had a lot of frustration about not being able to read. Like most teenagers, I was still learning to deal with my emotions. Part of growing up for me was learning to handle my anger. Most of us do one of two things with our anger. Either we act in or we act out. If we act in, we are quiet about our anger. We tend to take it out on ourselves. Masking the fact that we are angry. In elementary school, I acted in. If I disappeared in the classroom and the teacher did not know I was there, I had done my job.

When I got to high school my hormones kicked in. I grew a couple of inches and I decided that I was going to act out. My parents took the brunt of my anger. I did not act out so much toward my friends because I did not want to lose them. I acted out with my parents because I knew they would always love me.

One day after this had been going on for a while, I walked into the house and Dad was standing in the kitchen. he said, "You are coming with me."

"Where are we going?" I asked.

"Your mom and I are worried about you," he answered.

"What do you mean?"

"Well, it's your attitude," he said. "Your mom and I have this friend, Dr. Ron. He is a psychologist and hypnotist. We think he can help you."

"Okay," I said. It was not as if I had any choice.

When we walked into Dr. Ron's office, the first thing he said to me was, "Rob, I hear you are angry."

"You bet I'm angry," I said.

"Well, what do you want to do with that anger?"

"I want to be angry," I shrugged.

Then he said something that amazed me. He said, "You can do anything you want with that anger. Anger is just energy."

That was the first time I had ever heard that and it blew my mind. Anger is just energy. You can do whatever you want with it. Dr. Ron just looked at me and said, "What do you want to work on while you are with me? What do you want to do with your anger?" I figured he expected me to say I wanted to work on something like my reading or my writing or my math, so I set out to do something different.

"I think I want to work on football."

"Football!" he said. "What do you want to work on about football?"

"The part of football I want to work on is that I am not any good and I want to be better. I am 4th string. I would like to do better."

"Okay," Dr. Ron said.

I could not believe this, so I asked, "But how is helping me in football going to make my education better?"

"What I am going to teach you will amaze you and it will make everything about you life better."

Heavy Visualization

I was interested in football for a couple of reasons. First, one of my teachers in grammar school had told my parents that I should participate in a sport in which I could be successful. She said that she had learning disabilities as a child and a wise doctor had given her mother the same advice. The teacher had become a very good tennis player and gone on to a successful life. My parents insisted that I pick a sport. I chose football. In middle school I was at best a mediocre football player. In fact, I detested playing football.

In high school, I changed my mind about football. I still hated it, but I wanted desperately to be on the team even though I weighed in at 150 pounds and would be competing against 250-pound, muscle-bound guys. Why did I want to play? One word: Acceptance. To me at that point, acceptance meant a letter jacket. The players dated the cheerleaders, were held in awe by their classmates, and often were given special treatment by teachers. That was enough for me. Football was my sport.

There were a couple of problems. One was my weight. Another was that I was not very athletic. Still, the rewards were too great for me to pass up.

So when Dr. Ron offered me the opportunity to get better at football, I jumped on it. He began by saying, "Rob, we need to define your problem. Then we need to define you solution."

"The problem is I am too small. I only weigh 150 pounds."

"So what is the solution?" he asked.

"I guess the solution is, I need to get bigger," I answered.

"And how do you do that?"

"I guess I need to get into the weight room and lift some weights," I told him.

"Okay," he said, "that is what we will work on."

I thought, "Great, this guy can come to the weight room with me and work out!" But Dr. Ron had other ideas.

He said, "You sit right there and we are going to work on your weightlifting." I sat down and he said, "We are going to do it through your mind."

I was disappointed. I had thought we were going to get some results. 'Oh, well. At least this will kill the hour with Dr. Ron,' I thought.

We started talking about weight lifting and he asked me if I knew how to do the perfect squat?

I told him I did. "How often do you do it that way?" He asked.

"It depends on how much weight is on there," I said. "Sometimes I don't do it right at all."

"I want you to do it right every time with me," he said. "You are going to do it in you mind and you are going to do it perfectly every time."

I thought, 'I can do that since there is no weight involved. I can do it in my mind perfectly.'

He asked me what the most weight I had lifted was in the last year and I told him. He had me put that much weight on the bar that I had pictured in my mind. Then he had me start to lift it. We practiced lifting that amount of weight perfectly.

Then he said, "What is your goal? How much weight do you want to be lifting?"

"I want to be lifting about 300 pounds," I answered.

"Okay, we will work on that." So we started adding weight, picturing each increment of weight as we worked our way up to 300 pounds.

Once Dr. Ron had taught me this technique, I did it for about six weeks. Then spring training started.

Everyone was allowed to come out for the team so the coach was not too surprised to see me. The first thing he said to me was, "We need to hit the weight room."

So we went to the weight room and I picked-up the previous year's maximum weight. I added more and more weight. By the time we started practicing in pads, I was squatting 350 pounds. I was still 150 pounds, but I was squatting 350 pounds.

I started to think that maybe Dr. Ron was onto something. Maybe you could actually use your mind to make a difference in your life. I liked this idea. If I could squat 350 pounds, maybe I could take this success and transfer it to something else. All of a sudden, I now believed in myself and thought, "I am going to be a starting member of the Heritage High School football team!"

The Magic

I started telling myself that every day, over and over. "I am going to be a starting member of the Heritage High School football team!" Once I started believing it, I started telling everyone.

Finally a couple of my friends said, "Don't you think you should tell the coach?"

"Good idea!" I said, and I did it.

"Really?" Coach said.

"Yes."

"What position were you thinking of starting at, Rob?" He asked thoughtfully, looking me up and down. "Quarterback?"

"No," I said.

"Receiver?"

"No."

"Well, what do you want to be?"

"Center," I said.

"Center?" Coach said. "That is not a glory position at all."

"Yeah, Coach, but I think I can do it." By then I was beginning to realize that if you think you can do something, you probably can. Most things are 90% mental fortitude"

"I've got a problem with you being the center," he said.

"What?" I asked innocently.

"We are in quad-A football, son! We are in the most recruited region in Georgia. If you are at center, the smallest man you will face this year weighs 225 pounds and the biggest man weighs 305 pounds. Rob, you weigh 150 pounds. They will eat you alive. You want to be the starting center, the anchor for the offensive line?"

"Yeah, coach, I think I can do it," I said undaunted.

My confidence must have impressed him.

"Okay, Rob, I will give you a chance," he said. I was still 4th string center, but coach had his eye on me. The only thing that had changed was that I was actually in shape to accomplish this goal. I was stronger, both mentally and physically, and I also figured that people would not see me coming because I was so small.

I played my heart out for the rest of spring training and at the end of it the coach walked up to me and said, "Rob, you did it. You got the ball to the quarterback more than anybody else did. You are the starting center for Heritage High this year."

Congratulations came at me from all directions from my parents, my siblings and my friends. I reveled in the praise. They all said that I must love football to get out there and play at 150 pounds and get beat up every day. Little did they know that I still hated football. I did not like putting on that heavy uniform, practicing in 90-degree heat, or constantly getting battered by the opposing linemen. When I went home tired and aching, I questioned why I was doing it. I thought sometimes that I must be insane.

But I had a goal. The goal was to be accepted. I would never earn acceptance through my academic powers. I had to find it in some other way. I thought again of those guys walking through the halls of Heritage High School with their letter jackets, and I found the strength to go on.

When I talk to CEO's today, I ask them, "What do you think is motivating your employees?"

Inevitably, they say, "Money." But the fact is that less than 1% of people quit their jobs over money. Some of the most successful people in the country often do not know what is motivating their employees. It is something far more important than money: acceptance, acknowledgment, desires to help. CEO's need to find out what motivates their workers.

At Heritage High, I was motivated by a piece of blue material with a big H on it. To me, that letter jacket meant acceptance. And I was going to get the jacket and acceptance like every other starting member of our team.

The Big Game

A week before the first game of the season, I was standing in the kitchen at home when my dad walked in.

The big game is this Friday, Rob. The Rockdale-Heritage game, the big rivalry."

There were only two high schools in the county at that time. I told him I knew the game was about bragging rights. He asked if I had seen the newspaper and told me that I should look at it. He flipped open the Rockdale Citizen to the sports page. There was a picture of the huge 275-pound nose guard for Rockdale High. He looked bigger than life. The caption read, "Mark's worst nightmare. Mark was my quarterback, the guy I was supposed to protect against this nightmare.

'This guy is going to kill me,' I thought. "I am going to be wearing a letter jacket, but they are going to have to bury me in it after the game." It was hard to think of a positive outcome at that point. I had a vision of myself lying in a hospital bed, bandaged from head to toe with a nurse asking me if I knew my name.

But I had come this far, so Friday night I ran bravely out on to the field. The stadium lights were blinding and our students cheered until they were hoarse. Everyone in the county must have been there. I started doing my jumping jacks, warming-up when the first bad thing happened. I looked up and the Rockdale team was coming out of their locker room. The nose guard was so big I could see him across the field at a great distance. Two

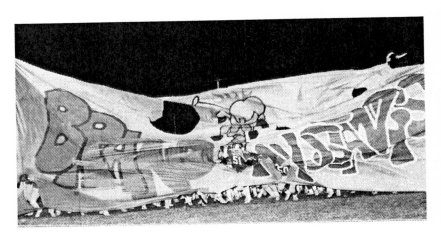

hundred and seventy-five pounds of vicious humanity came toward me. His thighs were so big that he waddled as he walked. I thought again of my impending doom.

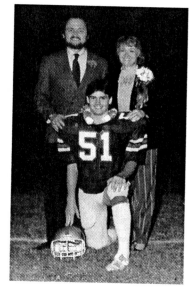

Then I came to my senses. I was committed. I had practiced the basics. I knew the steps. I had paid my dues. I could do this. No one was going to stop me but myself. I also realized that I had a powerful tool. I could visualize what I needed to do with this guy. I could do something "within" when I was "without." I started picturing in my mind what I could do to this nose guard. I could trip him. That is all I really had to do. If I could trip him every single play, I could keep him from getting to either Mark or me!

By the time the whistle blew, I was ready. When the first quarter came to an end, Rockdale was winning 7-0. When second quarter came to an end, we were on their tails with a score of 7-6. More importantly, the nose guard had not touched my quarterback. During halftime the coach gave us a "win one for the Gipper" speech. Our aching bodies responded with reserves of energy that we did not know we had. This game was important. We played above our skill level. By the end of the third quarter, we were leading 14-7. We could taste victory. In the fourth quarter the fans were on their feet, the score was 14-14. My quarterback scored the winning touchdown. We won the game and the bragging rights. Final score 21-14.

When I tell this story in elementary schools, I ask the kids, "How many tackles do you think this guy got?" They start saying a million. But the answer was zero. He did not get in on any tackles, not during the entire game. I was on the road to success, on the road to believing in myself.

The next week the coaches had voted me Offensive Player of the Week. I got a little plaque from the Village Inn Pizza. The 150-pound center had blocked out the 275-pound nose guard.

It was a great year. I got my letter jacket. I was popular and I was in heaven.

Dr. Ron had taught me something that all of us can do but few of us use: YOUR BRAIN. The fact is that you can get anything you want if you put the right information in your brain and give it enough energy. The other lesson I learned from this experience was, "play to your strengths."

I knew I could get the ball to the quarterback and I knew I could trip that nose guard. I did not try to play the glory positions of quarterback or wide receiver. I did not try to drive the nose guard to the ground. I did what I knew I could do well.

I won my battle for self-esteem. This success might not appear to have anything to do with my learning disability, but it did. My mind said that if I could succeed in football with no talent, I could use the same techniques to succeed in other areas of my life. Success breeds success. And that is when my real success began. I had learned that people can be happy and successful without being able to read and without knowing how to multiply.

Helping Others

I also learned that when you succeed, you have to share your success with others and help those who come after you. Notice that I don't say "it is a good idea to do this," or "you might try it." I believe it is essential. Here is how I found out about helping others:

I got my letter jacket my junior year and the next year I was actually walking down the hall at Heritage High with respect, doing what I wanted. I was dating the girls I wanted to date. I was having pretty much everything I wanted. My dream had come true.

Then one day a teacher walked up to me and told me about one of her students. She said he was leaving school crying every day and she did not know why. She asked if I could come to her class 6th period and see if I could figure out what was wrong with him. She explained that she had thought of me because many students looked up to me because of my football success and she knew I struggled in school. She said the student was learning disabled and hoped that I could help.

Did I have to do this? No. Should I have done it? Absolutely. With success comes responsibility.

I told her I would come to her class and began to walk away. She stopped me and said, "Wait a minute. There is something we want to do for you. The faculty knows that you wanted a certain English teacher that you did not get. If you do this for us, we will make sure you get that teacher." English was my worse subject and I needed a good teacher, so this was music to my ears. I thought this was a win-win situation. There was no way to lose in this one.

Sixth period rolled around and I went to class. In two days I figured out the problem that had eluded the teachers all quarter. The reason I could see it when they could not was this: It was not happening when the teacher was looking. It was the oldest, simplest scenario in the world. Three bullies. Three guys were picking on this learning disabled kid because he was a little slower and a little different from everybody else in the class. And these three guys were considered very cool.

All of a sudden, this situation was not a win-win; I did not like my role in it one bit. I had worked hard to get the social position I had and now I had been forced to jeopardize that position with these guys. I went home that night and thought about it. I had to do the right thing. I was accountable. I was accountable to myself and to the universe. "The universe will take my letter jacket back if I don't do something good with it."

So I figured out what might work to repair the situation. I practiced it in my head that night. (I only had one night to study for this test.) The next day, I went to the class and sure enough these guys started picking on the student again. It was a construction class and he was trying to build a little shelf. They started to move in on him.

I had thought about this moment all night long. The minute they went after him I knew what to do. If you have practiced something in your mind, your mind does not know that you have not actually accomplished it before. Your mind does not distinguish between things you have visualized and things you have actually done. Visualizing is just like practicing things in physical reality.

Before any of them knew what was happening, I stepped right into the group. I felt like I was almost outside my body. I said calmly but firmly, "Hey, we are not going to pick on him anymore!"

They looked at me with surprise and one of them asked, "What do you care?"

"What do you mean?" I asked.

"Why do you care what happens to him?" I had to think about that but the answer came quickly.

"Because I know how hard school is. I know how hard it is being a little different if you learn in a different style. That's all. That does not make you stupid. And I know that what we are doing is not right." I included myself in their group to win them over faster.

By the end of the day, they had decided that not only would they be friends with me, but that we would all be friends with the learning disabled student. I had solved the problem that easily.

When you have success in life, and you will, I challenge you to do something good with it. That is how to keep it and pass it on.

I learned a lot in high school but I was about to take on a whole new challenge. I was about to move up a huge step on the educational ladder without my mom nearby to support me.

CHAPTER 4

An Advocate for Myself: College

By the time I got to West Georgia College in 1986, I understood my learning styles and knew exactly what I needed in order to succeed in the educational system. What I did not know was whether or not the college administration and faculty would cooperate and provide for these needs. No formal programs for the learning disabled were available at that time.

Note to the instructor:

It is only recently that the area of Learning Disabilities has come to the attention of college faculties, because it is only recently that students with learning disabilities have begun to attend college. It is for this reason that this collection of materials related to learning disabilities has been assembled for teachers at West Georgia College who have a learning disabled student in a class.

Our major goal is to provide a support system for teachers who encounter these learning problems in students previously identified as having a learning disability. The services included in this system are detailed in the enclosed Accommodations for learning disabled students at West Georgia College.

If there is any way I can help, please contact me.

Dr. Ann Phillips, counselor
Coordinator of Special Services
 for Disabled Students
Student Development Center
136 Mandeville Hall
(ext. 416)

I knew that college-teaching styles depended strongly on reading and writing, and did not include the styles in which I learned. It was unsettling at first for my mother to be back in Conyers and away from me. I had to deal with things on my own now. I knew my mother had trained me well and her attitude naturally kicked in, the attitude of getting what I needed to learn today. I emulated my mother's attitude and got my education.

The Wheelchair Form

I had learned early how important it was to let people help and support me. Dr. Ann Phillips, the Director of Student Services at West Georgia, gave me a wonderful opportunity to do just that. Dr. Phillips was once asked why she was so eager to help me. She replied that it was her job. She never felt it was anything extraordinary. She may not have thought it to be extraordinary but it was.

Before my first quarter in college, Mom, Dad and I sat down with Dr. Phillips and discussed my strengths and weaknesses. Mom gave her chapter and verse about my history, my disability, and my requirements. We wanted to develop an official document listing the accommodations I needed in order to succeed. We hoped the documentation would make administrators and professors more likely to provide them.

The next step was deciding how to present this to the professors in a way that they could understand. The problem was, that at that time, people had a lot of assumptions about students who were learning disabled. If a blind or deaf student walked into the classroom, the teacher would not assume they were dumb. It would be obvious that the blind person would need to learn in an auditory way and that the deaf person would need to learn visually, but they would not be considered to be stupid and they would not be suspected of looking for a free ride. Although someone like me, who could see and hear and who appeared normal but had an auditory-visual learning style was often considered "dumb."

We looked for precedents and found one in an unlikely place, the Wheelchair Accommodation Form. Schools accept that students in wheelchairs have a physical disability. At that time, dyslexia was not considered a physical disability. However, Dr. Phillips, my mother and I thought of it as an "invisible physical disability." When dyslexia is defined this way, adapting the Wheelchair Accommodation Form to meet my needs made sense. The professors were used to seeing the physical disability form and that was to our advantage. We simply wrote my strengths and weaknesses on that form and listed the accommodations I would need.

"Give this to your professors the first day of class," Dr. Phillips said.

Again, we were using a three-step formula for getting what I needed as a learning disabled student: Communication, Learning Styles and Precedents. We communicated what I needed, described the learning styles that would need to be accommodated and used old precedent to set ones of our own by adapting the existing form to accommodate a learning disability.

Dr. Phillips believed in me and became my ally. She played a major role in my success in college. Throughout my years at West Georgia, she and I plotted, planned, and formed strategies. She told me that I was the first student who had ever received accommodations based on being learning disabled. They simply had not dealt with it up to that time. I was not the first diagnosed learning disabled student to go to the school, but I was the first who was accommodated. In that sense, Dr. Phillips and I were acting as pioneers.

Report Date: Oct. 2, 1989
Ann Phillips, Coordinator
Disabled Student Services

Student Disability Report
Student Development Center
West Georgia

Student's Name: Rob Langston   **SS✱**

Date First Enrolled: Sept. 1986   **Hours Earned At WGC: ⬛**

Advisor: Hunsicker   **Major:** Business, marketing

Kind Of Disability: Learning Disability: dyslexia.

General Description of This Student's Disability: Rob scrambles and reverses letters; it is very difficult for him to decipher the written word, so his reading is extremely slow and limited, although his intelligence is average or above. It is also very difficult for him to translate into writing what he hears.

How The Disability Affects This Student In Class Or On Campus:
1. Rob reads and writes very slowly in spite of having attended special classes from 3rd to 8th grade to teach him reading by phonics. The slowness in speed and recognition reduces his comprehension.
2. His spelling is very poor.
3. His writing is so slow as to be a distraction for him when taking notes.
4. Time limitations on a test are more nervewracking for Rob than for the average student.

Accommodations In Class Or On Campus That Can Aid The Student In Reaching The Standards And Requirements Of His Courses:
1. The slowness of Rob's reading and writing will necessitate <u>oral testing, testing apart from the rest of the class,</u> and <u>special timing</u> for a fair evaluation of his learning. Arrangements for oral testing or specially timed testing can be made by using a graduate student or by contacting Francie Burns, Director of Testing, ex. 6435, who is already aware of Rob's situation.
2. Please allow use of a tape recorder for note-taking situations.
3. <u>He is using taped textbooks whenever possible, and is using readers when tapes are unavailable.</u>
4. Where in-class writing is required, please allow extra time for slow writing and proof-reading.
5. Rob may need to check spelling of new terms with you after class. Writing terms and names on the board will help.

6. It would help for his instructor to experiment with different ways of testing him, and different ways of letting him write his papers, so he can show what he is capable of doing apart from areas affected by the learning disability.
7. The use of a calculator in math classes would be beneficial.

Strengths Available To This Student To Help Offset Effects of Disability:

1. Very strong auditory comprehension. Pays very close attention in class.
2. High ability in abstract and conceptual thinking and performing.
3. High ability in practical areas.
4. Is organized.

If you have questions or wish further information, please call Ann Phillips at Ext. 6428, Student Development Center.

69

By my third year, we had everything in place and the wheelchair form had been adapted to the student disability report shown earlier in this chapter. Today, it does not take that long. Institutions of higher education are adapting more and more to accommodate learning-disabled people. However, it is still important to be your own advocate. Many students do accept the role of self- advocate at different times in their careers based on their personalities, confidence, and level of maturity. Some may never assume this role. It is up to parents to set the example and support the student in becoming a self-advocate.

I learned by doing and watching my mother be my advocate for the first twelve years of my education. In college, I developed what I called the "blue collar approach" to being a self-advocate for the accommodations I needed. Basically, this involved doing whatever it took to get accommodations that were not freely provided by the school system.

My Blue Collar Approach

Nobody knew much about accommodations for learning disabled students so I went about getting them one-by-one in whatever way worked best. I made it up as I went along. This was my "blue collar approach." Whenever the system said that something could not be done, I demonstrated that it was possible. The "blue collar approach" requires confidence and an attitude of not being denied. You have to discard traditional thinking and begin thinking outside the box.

These are some of the accommodations I received using the 'blue collar approach."

1. Pre-Registration: Getting the Best Teachers

I embarked on a systematic search for the "best" teachers. To me that meant the teachers who cared. I had learned early that not every teacher could teach me. It took a special teacher and that teacher only had to have one quality. He or she had to care.

To find these special teachers, I first surveyed other students. I would say, "Who is the best English teacher at West Georgia?" After collecting many opinions, the names of one or two teachers usually surfaced as the "best." Then I just walked into the best teachers' offices, handed them my wheelchair form and said, "Hi, I am Rob Langston and I have dyslexia. I hear you are one of the best English teachers at West Georgia and I want to take you class in the fall. Here is my form telling you everything I will need: Note taker, reader, separate testing classroom, oral testing, etc."

At this point, even the best teachers were panicking. They were thinking, 'this student is going to be too much trouble.'

Then I hit them with my ace, "And here is what I will do for you." I gave them a list of things I would do for them if they would take me into their class. That list included:

I will attend every class. (If I do not show up for class, send someone to check on me because something is wrong.)

I will come to class prepared, having listened to and studied the materials.

.I will participate fully in class discussions.

I will always give 100% and do my best.

If I get behind, I will get a tutor.

This was my declaration that learning is a two-way street and a two-way responsibility. I was willing to do my part. How could a teacher turn away such a dream student? Very few said "No."

Then I would say, "I know I am asking for your syllabus an entire quarter in advance, and I know that could be a hardship on you if it is not fully prepared. The reason I am doing this is that I am going to have every assignment read onto tape so I can listen to it. And when you assign Machievell in the class to be read next week, guess what? I am going to pull my tape out and listen to it on the trip from Conyers to Carrolton and back. And when I come into your class, I am going to participate. My hand will always be up. I get 85% of what I know from listening and I will listen to the material for your class."

I didn't always get the teachers I wanted. I had picked my teacher, talked to the teacher, gotten the syllabus and went to the registrar's office to register for class. Still one problem was that I didn't always get the class because the class was full. At the time I was a self-advocate and didn't know what to do. I thought I'd do what I had always done, I'd call my mom. I asked what should I do since I didn't get the class and mom said, "just go to the class." I said, "I can't go to the class because I won't get credit for it if I'm not on the roll call".

But mom asked, "what's important, getting credit or learning?"

I answered, "I guess learning."

Mom said, "Then go to class."

I started the process of officially adding and dropping courses; in the meantime, I would go to the first day of the "best" teachers' classes even though I was not registered with them. I would sit in the front row and participate. If they asked me why I was there, I would give my talk about finding the best teachers. My next step was to wait out the one or two-week drop/add process to see if I could replace someone who had dropped the class. Most of the time no one would drop the class. After all, these were the best teachers. By the end of drop-add, I was a class fixture! No teacher ever threw me out of class because I was not officially enrolled. Instead, they raised the class limit by one. I then worked hard not to disappoint the teacher.

Dr. Phillips knew that I was interviewing my teachers and choosing the best ones and she was impressed with my efforts. She decided to take the process one step further by giving me permission to pre-register for all my classes. This would give me a much better chance of getting the teachers I wanted. I had an easier time getting this accommodation because I had already set the precedent of interviewing teachers with my "blue collar approach," and people saw that I was willing to do a lot of footwork myself. Administrators and teachers knew that I was willing to go the extra mile.

By the time I left West Georgia College, we had a running list of the best teachers. The teachers who had worked with learning disabled students in a positive way. This was a legacy to help others.

2. Note Takers

Another accommodation that was important to me was to have a note taker in each class. During college, I took a test that showed that my visual-auditory learning was on the level of a twenty-five year old. On the same test, I scored on a fourth grade level in my ability to spell what I was hearing.

Note taking was a nightmare for me. I could sit in class listening to the professor and collect most of the information out of the air on an adult level. But as I tried to write down what I had heard, I was committing it to paper on a fourth grade level. I was actually losing most of the information as I wrote in my slow, deliberate manner. Also, I would never be able to read the notes. The teacher kept talking and I listened less and less. I was trying to write what he or she had just said and missing what was being said next. My testing showed that I needed to sit in class and listen in order to absorb information. Taking notes interfered with that process.

In high school, the teachers would give me their notes to study so I could focus on listening. I had set a precedent to receive another accommodation in college. Even with the precedent set, I had to go about the accommodation the "blue collar" way.

I would go into the classroom the first few days and see who was taking the most notes. Then I would approach them after class. I introduced myself and explained my disability. I complemented them on their note taking and offer to pay them for copies. My offer was $20.

There is no law or reason you cannot pay students for their notes from class and there is no college student who is going to turn down $20 for doing something they had to do anyway. I told Dr. Phillips about the arrangement and she thought a note taker was a reasonable accommodation.

The school then provided me with note takers. On the first day of a new class, it became standard for the teacher to ask the class who was the best note taker. A few students would raise their hands, thinking they would get "brownie" points. The teacher would ask one student to stay after class. At the close of the lesson, the teacher, the volunteer and I would stay after class to talk. The teacher would explain the situation and ask the student to copy his or her notes after each class. Inevitably, the teacher would offer some reward such as extra credit to the cooperative student.

If the teacher did not help or if there were no volunteers, I put my "blue collar" approach into effect. I would find a student who wanted to make a few dollars and pay him or her to help me. Usually the note taker also became my study partner, creating a win-win for both of us.

3. Readers

When Dr. Levinson diagnosed me with dyslexia, I had automatically gotten access to the Library for the Blind[3]. I could get all my books on tape. I was grateful for that, but I realized early that my professors would assign the reading out of order and sometime only a few pages at a time. Having the entire book on tape was often not useful. I spent many frustrating hours trying to find the correct lesson on the tape. Today, the RFB&D (Recording for the Blind and Dyslexic) have new technology that allows you to listen to specific pages out of a book at the touch of a button.

My "blue collar" approach was to ask the teacher for the class syllabus and ask another student to read the assigned readings on to tape for me. Often my readers recorded over twenty tapes of information. They were flattered to be asked and appreciated the few dollars I gave them along with my gratitude. Generally, I had female readers because my mother and sister served as my models.

4. Calculators and Franklin Speller™

Another accommodation I was given was a calculator. My brain was not capable of learning the multiplication tables. Therefore, beginning in third grade, I was allowed to use a calculator.

The Franklin Speller™ was another of my accommodations. You give this tool the phonetic spelling of a word, and the speller gives you the correct spelling. If you come vaguely close to the correct spelling, the speller identifies and spells the word correctly for you. I was fortunate that I had learned phonics during the many years of tutoring and extra classes. The ability to use phonics allowed me to use the Franklin Speller™.

5. Alternative Class Lists

I was moving along steadily toward my degree, but one thing stood in my way: Foreign Language. Since I could not conquer English; there was little chance I was going to learn a foreign language.

If you run into a class you cannot pass, what do you do? You get an alternative class. That is what I did with foreign language. I was given a list of twenty alternative classes I could take to fulfill the foreign language requirement. The alternatives were studies of foreign history and cultures. I took two classes from the schools list and then the Georgia Board of Regents came out with an official list of alternative classes. There were only eight classes on the official list. I panicked. The new list did not include the classes I had already taken. I called to ensure my credits would count toward graduation, and the "inflexible" university wrote a letter saying the two classes I had taken would in fact count toward graduation. I still had to take two classes from the official Regents' list.

West Georgia College

Carrollton, Georgia 30118-0001
A SENIOR COLLEGE IN THE UNIVERSITY SYSTEM OF GEORGIA

OFFICE OF THE VICE PRESIDENT
404 836 6445

April 15, 1993

M E M O R A N D U M

TO: Registrar

FROM: The Vice President and Dean of Faculties

SUBJECT: Substitution for Language Requirement
          for Robert W. Langston,

I am authorizing the substitution of 20 hours of foreign culture courses listed below
for the foreign language proficiency requirement in the B.F.A. degree program for
Robert W. Langston,

      ENG 295   Ancient and Medieval Literature
      HIS 315   Near East in the Middle Ages
      HIS 416   Modern France
      HIS 445   Twentieth Century Europe

ENG 295 and HIS 315 were approved by Dr. Richard Dangle, Dean, School of Arts
and Sciences, prior to his retirement last June, even though these courses are not on
the approved institutional list of language substitutions.

Attached is the documentation of Mr. Langston's learning disability, indicating that
any further attempt of a foreign language with modifications would be futile.

ph

Enclosures

CC: Dr. Ann Phillips

     Mr. Robert W. Langston

This was an exercise of patience, persistence and perseverance.

Coping with Obstacles

I could not always get the professors to agree to accommodate my learning styles. One experience stands out as a "character building moment" for me. I went to Dr. Phillips and asked her to recommend an English teacher who might help me even though I was not in his or her class. I wanted a good English teacher to correct the punctuation and grammar on an essay for my primary English teacher. My primary English teacher agreed with Dr. Phillips that concepts are infinitely more important than grammar and punctuation, but I wanted to turn in a paper of which she would be proud.

Dr. Phillips referred me to a particular professor. I showed up in his office with my wheelchair form in hand to explain my disability and situation. He was the consummate professor, a short, round, balding man wearing glasses and holding a pipe in one hand. He sat behind the wooden desk surrounded by books in his cluttered office.

I explained my situation and asked him to help me correct the punctuation and spelling so I could turn in a perfect paper to my teacher. I had all the information. I needed help perfecting it.

He looked me straight in the eye and said, "I believe that learning disabled people are slow and lazy. Not only will I not help you do this paper; I would appreciate it if you never take my class. I am not the teacher for you."

I looked back at him and thanked him for his time agreeing that he was not a teacher for me. Then, I walked out.

He was right. I felt sorry for him and I was grateful that I had learned all the lessons I had learned. To withstand that kind of interaction, you have to have a level of confidence and belief in yourself. You have to know that it is the other person's sense of self worth, not your own, in question.

This would have previously shattered my self-esteem. I had created enough successes by this time to build a firm, strong, healthy concept of myself. I had learned not to allow anyone to influence who I was or what I could do. My confidence and self-esteem were now puncture-proof. I renewed my search for a teacher who would help and went back to Dr. Phillips. She gave me another professor's name and never recommended the first professor to another learning disabled student.

You do not have to associate with people who try to bring you down. Stay focused on what you need.

Looking for Success

I knew from playing football in high school that it was important to experience success in areas outside the classroom. When I entered college, I looked for an activity in which I could chalk up successes. I decided it would be pushing my luck to try college football. I noticed fraternity men got attention and I decided to ride a fraternity's coattails to success. With my older brother's help and with great excitement, I became a pledge at the Pi Kappa Alpha Fraternity.

I was a member for only a short time when to my dismay; the fraternity went into a nosedive. By my 3rd year of college, the intramural teams were virtually winless, the fraternity was $14,000 in debt and membership had dwindled down to only twenty members. One day a group of the members came to me and said, "Rob, we want you to be the president of Pi Kappa Alpha."

I can tell you, I was not overwhelmed with joy. I was not flattered nor was I honored to be singled out to run this dysfunctional organization. I went over in my mind all the things that were wrong with the fraternity. Then, I realized I was doing to them what people had done to me all my life. They had told me it could not be done. With that awareness, I accepted their offer and proclaimed not only would I be president, but within a year we would be the best fraternity on campus.

I do not remember their response. I am sure it was full of doubt and sarcasm. I immediately put my success attitude into motion and applied all the principles I had learned into changing the fraternity. The first thing I did was to get each member involved by appointing him to a committee and expecting him to be successful.

Within one year, we had expanded to 100 members, had completely paid off the $14,000 debt. We went undefeated in flag football, basketball, softball and soccer. Pi Kappa Alpha went from worst to first on campus in only one year. That year we won the first chapter award in ten years, The Havery T. Newell Award for the Most Improved Chapter in the nation! I was honored as one of twelve men out of 10,000 undergraduates nationwide for my service to the fraternity. Later that same year, I was inducted into the Order of Omega; an honor reserved for the top 3% of all fraternity and sorority members in the country.

How was I able to accomplish this? I believed that it could be done. My mother had taught me to believe that anything is possible and I had numerous experiences confirming that it was true. Next, I convinced others that it could be done with their help. We set the goal, took action, and marched forward with confidence.

Because of our attitude of success we attracted success.

Part 3: Getting What You Need

CHAPTER 5

What is Dyslexia?

Now that you have heard my story, I want to get down to the nuts and bolts of surviving and thriving with a learning disability.

"Learning disability" is a phrase used to describe a disability that interferes with the ability to process, store and/or retrieve information. Dyslexia is one of many learning disabilities. It is a term that has been around for a long time. The word dyslexia comes from the Greek words "dys" meaning poor or inadequate and "lexis" meaning words. It is characterized by problems in reading, listening, writing, speaking and/or math. I have heard it described as the circuitry for reading being short-circuited. That makes it more difficult for dyslexics to translate written words into sound. Both adults and children can have dyslexia. The problem can be subtle and hard to recognize or it can be pronounced and easy to identify.

We are still learning about dyslexia. We do know that it affects 10% to 25% of the population or more than 25 million people. We also know that it is a physical disability not a mental one. It is an invisible physical disability. This invisibility makes dyslexia hard for observers to understand.

How Dyslexia Works

The proof that dyslexia is a physical disability comes from using Magnetic Resonance Imaging (MRI). The neurological systems of people with dyslexia are wired differently from others, perhaps because of a problem with brain chemistry.[4]

To read successfully, the language center at the back of the brain and the visual-processing center in the forebrain must function together efficiently. The path between these sections must be clear and direct. In normal readers, this neuro-linguistic path is well defined and the information travels at a uniform speed. In dyslexics, the activity in the language center shows decreased activity while the activity in the part of the brain linked to spoken word is increased. MRI results show many more areas of the brain lighting up than lit up in the group of normal readers. This means that information does not travel at uniform speeds. When information takes this kind of scattered path, traveling randomly along different paths at varied speeds and out of the proper sequence, then it becomes difficult for us to process written information.

Here is how it works in practical terms. Suppose the teacher writes C-A-T on the board. My eyes take in the information and direct it to the reading/language center. My eyes focus on the "C" first and it begins a path to my reading center in the back of the brain. That "C" may take a very circuitous route through many areas of my brain delaying the arrival at the reading center. Meanwhile, my eyes have grabbed the "A" and it has started back to the reading center by an entirely different route, at a different speed. Finally, the "T" begins the path and makes a beeline for the reading center. Arriving out of breath, it looks around and finds none of the fellow letters have arrived. The "T" awaits the arrival of the "A" that positions itself following "T." Finally, the "C" arrives and stands at the end of the line. We now have all the letters that make up C-A-T, but they actually spell T-A-C. Because each letter has traveled a different path, at different speeds, the word C-A-T has been disassembled and reordered to form T-A-C.

The Dyslexia Institute says that dyslexia is a neurological problem of the brain communicating with itself. Dyslexic symptoms are not a result of laziness, lack of motivation, or psychological or social problems. In fact, many dyslexics are highly creative and show special talent in areas such as art, drama, music, electronics, athletics or architecture.

Scientists have isolated genes that they suspect are responsible for dyslexia. Researchers studying three generations of families with reading disorders have found a genetic basis for the condition. Although extensive research into the cause of dyslexia continues, no cure has been found. For that reason, we must accept that the problem exists, diagnose the symptoms, and find a solution that allows dyslexic children to be educated.

Are You Dyslexic?

After accepting that the problem exists, the next step is identifying the people who have dyslexia. This search is not easy because each dyslexic person's problems are different in scope and in severity.

Most children with dyslexia are not identified until they enter school. Problems with reading, writing, math and other schoolwork surface drawing attention to the issue. A family history of learning disabilities should put parents on the alert to watch out for dyslexic symptoms, but many children are only mildly affected and may be diagnosed only after they have begun to fail at school. Unfortunately, these children are often thought to be unmotivated, lazy or dumb.

Some of the characteristics indicating dyslexia are:

- Family members who are slow readers
- Difficulty in quickly determining right and left
- Lack of coordination
- Poor organizational skills
- Speech problems
- Reversal of letters or words when writing
- Short attention span
- Delayed spoken language
- Difficulty in expressing thoughts orally
- Problems following stories read from books
- Inability to follow sequential instructions

A person with dyslexia may have one, none or many of these characteristics. Dyslexia is usually more prevalent and more severe in boys than in girls[5]. It occurs in people with all levels of intelligence, although more often in average or above average learners.

More Clues

The Dyslexia Institute (www.Dyslexia-inst.org.uk). lists the following clues for recognizing a person with dyslexia:

ALL AGES:

- Is he bright in some ways with a "block" in others?

- Is there anyone else in the family with similar difficulties?

- Does he have difficulty carrying out three instructions in sequence?

- Was he late in learning to talk or speak clearly?

AGES 7-11:

- Does he have particular difficulty with reading or spelling?

- Does he put figures or letters the wrong way, for example 15 for 51, 6 for 9, b for d, "was" for "saw?"

- Does he read a word and then fail to recognize it later on the page?

- Does he spell a word several different ways without recognizing the correct version?

- Does he have a poor concentration span for reading and writing?

- Does he have difficulty understanding time and tense?

- Does he confuse right and left?

- Does he answer questions orally, but have difficulty writing the answer?

- Is he unusually clumsy?

- Does he have trouble with sounds in words, example poor sense of rhyme?

AGES 12-ADULT

- Is he sometimes inaccurate in reading?
- Is his spelling poor?
- Does he have difficulty taking notes or copying?
- Does he have difficulty with planning and writing essays, letters or reports?

If you answer "yes" to many of the above questions, you may want to get professional advice. If your child answers "yes," you should get advice as soon as possible. Early diagnosis is the first and most important step. If there is no intervention before the third grade, the majority of those affected will have the problem for the remainder of their lives.

After diagnosis, the next step is to provide the child with a multi-sensory learning environment with specially trained teachers who understand his unique learning style. Every child has a right to learn and the law is on our side. It requires the schools to provide for all children's needs.

What is Next?

We know dyslexia does not reflect low intelligence, lack of motivation, mental problems or lack of opportunity. More and more studies suggest that we may one day find a cure for dyslexia. Until a cure is found, accommodations are the only answer for creating an environment in which students with dyslexia can learn. Only testing can establish a student's disability, only through official results will accommodations be given by the school system. That is why the next two chapters are on accommodations and testing. Put them to use for you so that you get the services you need.

Dyslexia is a learning disability. It is not a sentence to ignorance or failure. It can be a catalyst for success and creativity.

CHAPTER 6

Getting the Accommodations You Need

When I was in school, my mother and I handled each situation as it came to us. We did not know what accommodation was needed until we were in the middle of the problem. When I told her, "I can't write what I know," we realized I needed oral testing. When I could not complete a test, even though I had unlimited time because the next class had gotten underway, we realized I needed a separate classroom. When I was losing most of what was said in class because I was struggling to take notes, I realized I needed a note taker.

What we did was hit-and-miss. You can get accommodations in a much more systematic way. Currently, there is more awareness about learning disabilities and we have better laws. You have only to put the information to use.

What is an Accommodation?

My definition of an accommodation is the help that each student needs to learn successfully. Dr. Ann Phillips, my advocate at West Georgia College, describes them as "the things that can be done that help set the disability aside so that the ability can be learned or shown or fairly evaluated, to keep learning disabilities from preventing students from learning or being tested fairly."

One of the dictionary's meanings is: "Aid, comfort, or convenience; willingness to help; obligingness; compliance."[6]

In essence, this means that an accommodation "evens the playing field." But definitions do not really matter. What matters is getting whatever it takes in terms of resources, tools and techniques in order to be successful in getting an education.

People said to me, "Anybody could have gotten through college with all those accommodations!"

I answered, "That is the point."

We should all go to college. We should all have what we need to be lifelong learners. If we train people to look for the accommodations they need as early as elementary school then teach and test the way they learn, we would have a better, happier, and more productive society. Bright, intelligent people would be productive citizens instead of depending on society to provide for them, or struggling on their own.

The Accommodations Formula: Communication, Learning Style, and Precedents

I have spoken of the three-step formula for getting accommodations. I have also described the path my mother and I took to put the formula into action while I was in school. When I speak to people today about accommodations, I take what we used and make it a very specific system for getting what one needs in order to learn. This simple formula is why I was successful in the educational system. Because of the system's importance

I will take the opportunity to look at the steps in more detail. With these steps, you can get any accommodation.

- COMMUNICATION
- LEARNING STYLE
- PRECEDENTS

Each step builds on the one before. Open communication defines the problem and leads to discovering your learning style. When you define your learning style (auditory, visual, kinesthetic, etc.) and use it successfully in the classroom, a precedent is set. Once the precedent for an accommodation is established, the school is required by law to provide it for you. Our legal system is based on precedents. Get a precedent set for an accommodation, show that you can learn that way, and by law the school has to give you that accommodation.

Each individual element of the formula is important although, communication, learning style, and precedents are also synergistic.

Communication

In my case, communication began between my mom and me when I told her, "I can't write what I know." That provided her with what she needed to know to get me what I needed. She could communicate with my teachers about my problem. Later, she taught me to communicate with them directly.

When I talk to students, I stress that they have got to stop hiding and talk to other people about their problems. If they do not, they cannot be helped. When I talk to teachers, I tell them the same thing. Often, teachers come to me after a program and ask for advice regarding a specific student. They say, "He is just like you. What should I do with him?"

"What does he say you should do?" I will ask. They look at me as if I was crazy.

"I have not asked him," is often the reply.

I tell teachers to listen to their students. Kids want to learn and have the answers on how to succeed. Who knows more about their learning styles, even when they are young, than the people trying to learn? My mother understood that.

When I came home from failing that test, she quizzed me. I told her I remembered the answers and repeated them to her. That gave her information and she had even more information when I communicated further with her. It was because of that communication that my mother decided I should be tested for what I knew and not what I could write.

The next step was for Mom to communicate with the teacher. She explained the problem and asked the teacher if she would give me credit if I answered the test questions orally. The teacher agreed. I proved to her that I knew the answers and showed that when tested a different way, I could succeed. Passing the test by speaking the answers instead of writing them, established my auditory learning style and oral testing became a precedent. That is how we completed the three steps of the formula.

Communication has to go on all the time between students and their parents, between students and their teachers and between parents and teachers. There is no progress without communication.

Learning Style

Communication is how to find your learning style. Everyone has a different learning style and some have more than one. We might learn in an auditory, visual or kinesthetic way. We may also learn using a combination of these styles.

I think that the learning preferences are in these ranges:

Visual: 29%

Auditory: 34%

Kinesthetic: 37%

By the time we are adults, we are so inundated with visual stimuli that the above percentages change resulting in the majority of adults being visual learners.

Wayne Dyer quotes learning styles research on his tape, *Improve Your Life Using the Wisdom of the Ages.* He talks about a group of students using the visual learning style.[7] Some of the students excelled and scored in the genius range. The same group of students was then tested using the auditory mode of learning. Again, some students excelled and scored in the genius range. However, it was a different group of students who excelled under this mode. The test was then given to the same students in the kinesthetic (experiential) learning style. Approximately the same number of students excelled, but again, it was a different group from those who had excelled in the previous tests. Dyer's conclusion is that there is a genius in everyone. We just need to know how to tap into that genius.[8]

Many experts in learning styles admit that some students will learn no matter how the material is presented. Others will learn an adequate amount to pass in one style, but will learn more if the lessons are presented differently. Still others are unable to learn if their learning style is different from the one employed in the classroom.

Dr. Ann Phillips often speaks of learning disabled students who fail in school. She believes that many of these students could be salvaged before they fall through the cracks. The solution is a program that is orientated to deal with learning disabilities in a proactive manner. We could reach out for these people, provide for them, and keep them achieving from the very beginning of their educational careers. Dr. Phillips also says that such technologies as computers and dictation machines are tremendous tools for helping these students.

Dr. Phillips had the opportunity to watch sixteen and seventeen-year-olds since they were four and five-years-old. These students were intelligent, sharp little children. Now, they have been left behind. They were students who could not learn in the traditional way and they came to believe that they were failures. They lost the promise of a bright future.[9]

There are many things that can be done to help learners. If you are a parent or a student, try different methods to find what learning styles work. Whenever you see a piece of the puzzle, grab it. If you are a teacher, look for pieces of your students' puzzles. Focus on cutting through the red tape and on the question, "How is this child going to learn today?" Remember, in order for a child to become a lifelong learner, he or she has to have self-esteem. Our society has ignored generations of students who learn in ways that are not traditional. It is not these children who have failed. It is our educational system.

Precedents

If you set a precedent, it is difficult for people to stop giving you what has been proven to work. When a precedent is used again and again, it becomes the rule instead of the exception. Then the accommodation is established. When this occurs, each and every student with a documented learning disability can ask for and receive the same accommodation.[10]

The reauthorization of IDEA (Individual Disability Education Act), passed in 1997, states that if the parent can show in the IEP (Individualized Education Plan) Group that a child learns better under certain conditions, the school must provide those learning conditions for the child.[11] After one teacher tested me orally, we could go to the next teacher and say, "Rob made a 20 on a written Science test, but when given the test orally, he scored a 92." This is the precedent that my parents could bring to an IEP Group. Under the current law, the school has to act on this information.

When I was in elementary school, my mother had never heard of IDEA or the IEP Group. But she did know that if she got an accommodation to work in one situation, it was easier to get it in the next situation. Her last words in every parent-teacher conference and after establishing each new precedent were, "I want it in Rob's permanent file."

This led to the crucial paper trail and the history that eventually got me the accommodations I needed. Each small step was documented and that lead to other small steps and another giant leap was accomplished.

The Parent's Role

Dr. Ann Phillips stresses how important it is for the parent or parents to come to the school and discuss their children's special needs. Many parents worry about being overly protective, but Dr. Phillips tells parents not to worry. She feels that all students, particularly learning disabled students, need their parents' help and support.

She encourages parents not to relinquish their child's cause when he or she becomes a freshman in college and then expect that he can immediately accept the role of advocate for himself. Students do not automatically become their own advocates after college arrival. Dr. Phillips believes that many will fail if you do not stay with them.

If parents drop the ball, students can start the downhill slide even before they get to college. This usually happens when parents believe that they do not have the right to ask for special concessions from the educational system. We often see the system as a huge, foreboding, unwavering monster, one that will shut us out unless we conform.

I think that when parents walk into a school, particularly in elementary school, they immediately become children again. The aroma of baked bread from the cafeteria, the long, bare hallway, and the noise of children being "sssh-ed" by teachers takes them back to their own childhood. In their minds, they shrink in size. The teacher once again becomes the authority figure that they are afraid to provoke. The principal is even more frightening.

My advice to parents is this: if you are afraid of the system, get over it. Many times, the accommodations I required to succeed in school did not seem reasonable. My mother always said "nothing is out of bounds when it comes to getting my child's needs served." She focused on what it would take for me to get through school and risked being laughed at because of her "ridiculous" requests. If you want your child to function at the highest level, you have to get them taught under the conditions that optimize their learning.

You need to be an advocate for your child. This does not mean you have to be rude or irrational. Although my mother demanded a great deal from the educational system, she also got many special arrangements through the "winning with honey" approach.

Recently, I was in a counselor's office waiting to talk to the students when a parent flew in demanding the counselor's attention. Before a single word came out of her mouth, I could tell she was angry. Her demeanor spoke volumes. She said to the counselor, "I need to talk with you right now." The counselor explained that it was time for her to introduce me to the school audience, so she did not have time at that moment. The woman insisted. I backed away from the desk, doing my best to look inconspicuous.

The first sentence from the parent was, "You are raising my child wrong." My mind reeled and I did not hear another word she said. I could not believe the parent felt the school should be raising her child. We cannot blame everything on the system. Ultimately, it is the parents' responsibility to make sure that children get the tools and accommodations they need to learn.

The Teachers' Part

Ideally, the parent is the advocate for the learning disabled child. Although, many children do not have a parent advocate. I challenge teachers to accept the advocate role for children who do not have a parent advocate. We live in a society with many single parent homes. If a teacher discovers one small piece of the learning puzzle for a child, the educational career of that child is changed forever. It may be the one thing that allows the student to succeed.

When you figure out a piece of a student's learning puzzle, grab it! Put it in the student's permanent file. It is the most powerful red tape cutter we have. Once it is there, it follows that child for the rest of his or her life. My mother grabbed every piece of my puzzle and held on to it for me until I was old enough to adapt it for myself.

Teachers tell me that they recognize what is needed to help a particular child, but they do not provide the accommodation because they do not know if it is right to do so. IDEA now says that it is not only right to provide the accommodation, it is required under law. Another reason teachers do not give the accommodation is that they are afraid of doing students a disservice. They feel the students eventually have to go out in the world and survive without accommodations. Therefore, they need to learn to do so now.

I say that getting these accommodations gives a child what is needed to survive, which is an education. The educational system is the process of getting them the training needed to go out into the world and be a productive person. Withholding accommodations because they might not be available later is a little like saying; I cannot use my calculator because I might not always have it by my side. I have a calculator at my desk, in my car, everywhere. They cost three dollars and I am willing to buy as many of them as I need, that is the real world.

On several occasions I have heard Phil Pickens, Director of the Department of Exceptional Children for the

State of Georgia, say, "If you (a teacher) are going to err, err on the side of the child or parent." I think he is exactly right.[12] All I ask is for the school system to level the playing field for the student with learning disabilities. These students do not need an advantage. They do need to be allowed to show what they know. I was appalled when a principal at a school where I spoke said, "I want you to talk with my teachers, but I do not want you to talk to the students' parents. They might get involved in their students' lives and cause problems at the school." Thankfully, this attitude is changing.

Dr. Phillips says that today, the State University of West Georgia is developing a special class for learning disabled students to tell them how to deal with college, how to take better notes, or how to get around not being able to write and listen at the same time. They are being told how to compensate for their disability and given tips on getting through college. She adds that West Georgia does provide tutoring for learning disabled students. The tutor appointed, is usually a good student but is not specifically trained to work with learning disabled students. Dr. Phillips believes that a teacher hired to work specifically with learning disabled students would be a valuable asset.

"Regular teachers simply do not have the time to learn how to work with learning disabled students," she says. As shocking as this sounds, Dr. Phillips says that the teachers would be the first to tell you this. It is not that they do not want to learn, but they have too much to do already. They are overworked preparing lessons and test, grading papers, meeting research requirements and publishing. Even for the most dedicated, committed teacher, there is little time for workshops, seminars and training classes. This magnifies the need for a teacher hired specifically to help learning disabled students. At most schools of higher learning, there is no room in the budget for such a teacher.

Each student is different and each requires his own unique combination of accommodations. That is why I encourage every student and parent to identify the students' learning styles and make sure the appropriate accommodations are provided. No one knows the students' needs better than the student and his parents.

Here are some accommodations I received. Use this as a starting point and add or delete as needed:

- Oral testing

- Separate classroom for test taking

- Untimed tests

- Readers

- Note takers

- Pre-registration

- Alternative classes

- Calculator

- Franklin Speller™

CHAPTER 7

Making Tests Work for You

In my early school years, tests were nightmares for me. Over the years, I learned to use them to my advantage.

Testing is your friend.

This has not always been my perspective. In fact, I dreaded testing for most of my school career. I was afraid of tests because they pointed out my inability and deficiencies.

Testing is scary for students and parents. My parents and I were never eager to hear the results. The scores reminded us of what I could not do because of my learning differences. I suffered from doing poorly, and they suffered from having their worse fears confirmed and seeing me suffer. I had to develop a thick hide, because no matter what my age, testing always was a tremendous emotional and mental stress for me. Each time I was tested, I had to gather up my self-esteem and start rebuilding again.

By the time I was last tested, I had a pretty healthy self-esteem and was within reach of hanging a degree on my wall. Still, the testing took a psychological toll. I spent three days with the testers, only to find that I had six strengths out of the twenty-two for which I was tested. I failed sixteen times out of twenty-two. When he asked me the definition of a word for which I could not verbalize the meaning, or when he asked me to follow written instructions and I could not, it was easy to slip into feeling like a failure. Although, the tester continued to assure me that it was okay not to know the answers, I walked out feeling very low and briefly questioned my true worth.

That is the bad news of testing. The good news is that I graduated from college because of testing. I could do that because I had learned something very important. I learned that the key to overcoming negativity about testing is keeping your focus on the rewards it can bring.

Focus on the Rewards

By focusing on the rewards and benefits that testing brought me, I was allowed to embrace the testing itself. I had also embraced my dyslexia as a gift. I began to shift my attention away from the discomfort and concentrate on the benefits I receive from testing.

Testing and documentation are essential and powerful tools. They help learning disabled students get what they need from the educational system. Testing leaves a paper trail. The value of this trail cannot be overemphasized. The educational system loves a paper trail. With each test and each result, the educational history carries more weight. It says: "Rob can do this, but he can not do that." That paper trail gets heavier and heavier and when the time comes to buck the system, the supporting information is available. "Rob gets a score of 20 without his accommodation and a score of 92 with the accommodation."

The documentation becomes your foundation for getting services and accommodations. Again, my mother said after every conference and after every precedent was established, "I want this in Rob's permanent file." The result of this persistence was possibly the largest permanent record in the history of Rockdale County Schools.

Testing is generally provided by the school system, but it is not always easily available. There are two problems. First, the school must recognize that the child has a problem. If the school does not see this, it is not interested in testing the student. Second, the waiting list for testing may be long. Several years may pass, as they did in my case, before testing is provided. Parents must find a way to have their child tested outside the system if the system does not provide what is needed.

Private testing is often the answer. Some parents worry that private testing will not mean anything to the school system or that it will not stand up under educators' scrutiny. This was not true in my case. When Dr. Levinson said I had dyslexia, the school system accepted it. Not only was my private testing accepted, but also it allowed me to receive accommodations. Private testing is most valuable when the parents determine ahead of time what the test needs to show in order to secure services for their child. You can then ask that the test be adapted to fulfill that need. My mother knew, for instance what she wanted confirmed from Dr. Levinson was a diagnosis of dyslexia.

If you go in with a solution and a specific request then both the testers and the educational system can provide the answers. When I had difficulties in school, I presented the solution instead of just griping about the problem. Most educators respected this and were willing to help.

Focus on Your Needs

Let the tests help you. Use them; do not let them use you. Focus on the parts of the test that will get you support, and do not feel compelled to tell everyone everything about the test.

When I scored 84 on an IQ test in second grade, my mother recognized that this was an inaccurate reflection of my mental abilities, and so she never told anyone this score. Learning disabilities were not understood at that time, so she was embarrassed to tell anyone for fear they would think that I was mentally deficient. Why did I score so low if I was smart? My score was low because the test was not designed to test my knowledge. It was geared toward people who were proficient in reading and writing. It proved only who was good at reading and writing.

After this IQ test, my mother wanted me re-tested. Finally, in the sixth grade, the system agreed to administer the IQ and skills test again. However, after three years of waiting, my mother knew she could not get the accommodations she wanted for me without test results showing that I had a learning disability. That is when my dad took me to Dr. Levinson.

In the ninth grade, the school system finally did test me. The staff recognized my learning disability, and they gave me the test that circumvented reading and writing skills. My true ability and intelligence were more accurately determined from performing these puzzle-type assembly tasks.

It was no surprise to my family that my IQ was in the superior/above average range, based on this new kind of test. I was the one who was surprised (and elated), given my history of failure in school. I had proof that I was bright, but simply had a learning disability. What a relief! What a boost to my self-esteem! From that time forward, I viewed both education and myself in a different light. The teachers saw me differently and revised their expectation of my potential for success. Research has proven that children live up to or down to expectations. This gift was priceless and it came to me through testing.

In the 12th grade, I was given a Psyche-educational Reevaluation. Included in this evaluation were the Wechsler Adult Intelligence Scale Revised (WAIS-R) and the Woodcock-Johnson Test of Achievement. On the WAIS-R, I again scored in the average range. The Woodcock-Johnson Tests pointed out my learning disabilities.

My score on Letter-Word Identification was grade 9.1. On Calculation, I was on a 7.4 grade level while slipping to grade level 4.9 on Dictation (Written Language Cluster). These scores did not matter to me or greatly affect my self-esteem. I was already well aware of my abilities and my disabilities. I had such a strong foundation that no test could convince me that I was not bright. There was one piece of information included in the testing results that was of importance to me. A statement in the Observations and Impressions section that read, "He is enthusiastic and eager about learning and expresses the wish to attend college after high school." I had become a life-long learner.

Climbing the Mountain

The first mountain I had to climb and overcome was the Scholastic Aptitude Test (SAT). To be accepted into college a student must make a certain score on this test. Each college and university has it's own score requirement. Most college-bound high school seniors have taken this test several times in order to improve their scores. Fortunately, my documented learning disabilities allowed me to take the SAT verbally, untimed, and in a separate classroom. I was the first person from my high school to take an oral SAT. Unfortunately, I was only allowed to take an oral SAT once. Even with my accommodations, I

CONFIDENTIAL

PSYCHOEDUCATIONAL REEVALUATION

ROCKDALE COUNTY SCHOOL SYSTEM

NAME: LANGSTON, Rob
AGE: 18 years, 3 months
BIRTHDATE: 11-28-67
PARENTS: Martha and Smoot Langston

DATE: 2-24-86
EXAMINER:
SCHOOL: Heritage High
GRADE: 12

REFERRAL AND BACKGROUND INFORMATION

Rob is enrolled in the resource Learning Disabilities program and was referred
for a three-year reevaluation. He is currently receiving support for regular
education classes for one period per day. He passed vision and hearing screenings
on 2-6-86. Rob has not repeated any grades. School attendance is good.

Consult the Psychological Services file for complete background information.
Recent and/or especially significant occurrences or data include the following:

> The LD resource teacher reports that IEP goals are being met totally.
> She states that "since Rob has been in the program, goals have been
> to provide avenues of compensation for his reading disability. This
> has proven to be effective. There has been growth in skills/confi-
> dence for reading and written language.

> On the Parent Questionnaire, the parents report that they are pleased
> with Rob's school progress. They state that Rob is doing better in
> school than ever before because of his oral work. However, Rob is
> still seen as a poor reader and terrible speller. They believe school
> personnel can be most useful in continuing his oral work, as well as
> continuing to teach him skills to compensate for his lack of reading
> and spelling skills.

OBSERVATIONS AND IMPRESSIONS

Rob is a handsome, alert, neatly groomed youth who worked very hard on all tasks
presented. His reading was very slow and laborious as material became more difficult. His speed was good and he showed confidence on puzzle-type, assembly tasks.
Rob said that he had forgotten much of his math. He said he felt he had memorized it
before without real understanding. His spelling suggested a phonetic approach.
Rob prefers to print and does so neatly. He is enthusiastic and eager about
learning - expresses the wish to attend college after high school.

TEST RESULTS AND INTERPRETATION

Wechsler Adult Intelligence Scale - Revised*
Verbal Scale score	105	Range - Average
Performance Scale score	108	Range - Average
Full Scale score	107	Range - Average

WOODCOCK-JOHNSON TESTS OF ACHIEVEMENT

NAME _Bill Johnston_   DATE _2-24-86_ ca _18-3_ 10 _/07_ (-15)_ _92_ (-20)_

	Grade Score	Instructional Range — Easy / Difficult	Age Score	Percentile Rank	Percentile Rank Range	Functioning Level*	Standard Score
Letter-Word Identification							
Word Attack							
Passage Comprehension							
READING CLUSTER	9.1	6.6 to 12.9(5)	14.4	26 at grade / 30 at age	21 to 31 at grade / 25 to 37 at age	BA at grade / BA at age	90 / 92
Calculation							
Applied Problems							
MATHEMATICS CLUSTER	7.4	6.3 to 9.0	12-10	10 at grade / 19 at age	4 to 14 at grade / 14 to 25 at age	MD at grade / MD at age	81 / 87
Dictation							
Proofing							
WRITTEN LANGUAGE CLUSTER	4.9	4.0 to 6.2	10-0	5 at grade / 8 at age	3 to 7 at grade / 6 to 10 at age	MD at grade / SD at age	75 / 79
Letter-Word Identification							
Applied Problems							
Dictation							
SKILLS CLUSTER		to		at grade / at age	to at grade / to at age	at grade / at age	

* VS – VERY SUPERIOR
S – SUPERIOR
AA – ABOVE AVERAGE
A – AVERAGE
BA – BELOW AVERAGE
MD – MODERATE DEFICIT
SD – SEVERE DEFICIT

109

For the Children

WAIS-R TEST RESULTS PROFILE

Confidential

CONFIDENTIAL

PSYCHOEDUCATIONAL REEVALUATION

Name _Rob Langston_   Age _18_   School _Heritage_   Grade _12th_

SCALED SCORES

ROCKDALE COUNTY SCHOOL SYSTEM

SUBTESTS Verbal Scale	DEFICIENT	BORDER-LINE	LOW AVERAGE	AVERAGE	HIGH AVERAGE	SUPERIOR	VERY SUPERIOR	SUBTEST MEANINGS
Information	1	2 3 4	5 6 (7)	8 9 10 11	12 13	14 15	16 17 18 19	Information from Experience and Education
Digit Span	1	2 3 4	5 6 7 8	(9) 10 11	12 13	14 15	16 17 18 19	Attention and Rote Memory
Vocabulary	1	2 3 4 5	6 7 8	(9) 10 11	12 13	14 15	16 17 18 19	Word Knowledge from Experience and Education
Arithmetic	1	2 3	4 5 6	7 (8) 9 10 11	12 13	14 15	16 17 18 19	Mental Arithmetic Concentration
Comprehension	1 2	3	4 5 6	7 8 (9) 10 11	12 13	14 15	16 17 18 19	Practical Knowledge and Social Judgment
Similarities	1	2 3	4 5	6 7 8 9 10 11	12 13	14 15	16 17 18 19	Logical and Abstract Thinking Ability

NAME: LANGSTON, Rob
AGE: 18 years, 3 months
BIRTHDATE: 11-28-67
PARENTS: Martha and Smoot Langston
EXAMINER:
SCHOOL: Heritage High
GRADE: 12th
DATE: 2-24-86

REFERRAL AND BACKGROUND INFORMATION

Rob is enrolled in the resource Learning Disabilities program and was referred for a three-year reevaluation. He is currently receiving support for regular education classes for one period per day. He passed vision and hearing screening 2-6-86. Rob has not repeated any grades. School attendance is good.

Consult the Psychological Services file for complete background information present and/or especially significant occurrences of data (include the LD data).

The LD resource teacher reports that IEP goals are being met totally. She states that "since Rob has been in the program, goals have been to provide avenues of compensation for his reading disability. This has proven to be effective. There has been growth in skills/confidence for reading and written language.

Performance Scale								
Picture Completion	1	2 3	4 5	6 7 8 9 10 11	12 13	14 15	16 17 18 19	Visual Alertness and Visual Memory
Picture Arrangement	1	2 3	4 5	6 7 8 9 10 11	12 13	14 15	16 17 18 19	Interpretation of Social Situations
Block Design	1	2 3	4 5	6 7 8 9 10 11	12 13	(14 15)	16 17 18 19	Analysis and Formation of Abstract Designs
Object Assembly	1	2 3	4 5 6	7 8 9 10 (11)	12 13	14 15	16 17 18 19	Putting Together of Concrete Forms
Digit Symbol	1	2 3	4 5	6 7 8 9 10 11	12 13	14 15	16 17 18 19	Speed of Learning and Writing Symbols

On the Parent Questionnaire, the parents report that they are pleased with Rob's school progress. They state that Rob is doing better in school than ever before because of his oral work. However, Rob is still seen as a poor reader and terrible speller. They believe school personnel can be most useful in continuing his oral work, as well as continuing to teach him skills to compensate for his lack of reading and spelling skills.

OBSERVATIONS AND IMPRESSIONS

Rob is a handsome, alert, neatly groomed youth who worked very hard on all tasks presented. His reading was very slow and laborious as material became more difficult. His speed was good and he showed confidence on puzzle-type, assembly tasks. Rob said that he had forgotten much of his math. He said he felt he had memorized it before — without real understanding. His spelling suggested a phonetic approach. Rob prefers to print and does so neatly. He is enthusiastic and eager about learning — expresses the wish to attend college after high school.

WAIS-R IQ

V _105_

P _108_   TEST RESULTS AND INTERPRETATION

FS _107_   Wechsler Adult Intelligence Scale – Revised*

Examiner _____

Date _2-24-86_

Verbal Scale score	105	Range – Average
Performance Scale score	108	Range – Average
Full Scale score	107	Range – Average

110

scarcely scored high enough to be accepted at West Georgia College. With the same score today, I would not have met the more stringent requirement.

In order to graduate from college when I was in school, every student was required by the State Board of Regents to take an exit exam to prove that he had satisfactorily mastered English. I sweated bullets over this one. A student's college degree would be withheld if he or she did not get a passing grade on the Regent's Testing Program Essay Test. For years, I had been taken out of English class to study phonics and reading. To this day, I know little grammar and have little experience with the written word.

The two essay questions from which I could choose were:

1. "In spite of advances in scientific knowledge, people are still superstitious." Agree or disagree.

2. "What situations are most stressful for you?" Discuss.

I selected the latter topic, the most stressful situation, and titled my essay, I Find It hard To Do Something I Do Not Know How To Do.

In the essay, I wrote that Reading, Writing, and English are the most stressful situations for me. English was the major stress. (Actually, writing the essay was probably one of the most stressful tasks I completed in school.) My essay contained many crossed out words because I was attempting to sound competent in English and vocabulary, and the punctuation was entirely guess-work. These tests were sent to three professors at various universities for grading. To my amazement, I passed. Either the educator grading the test took pity on me because I wrote about my disabilities, or the grading was very lenient.

For the Children

REGENTS' TESTING PROGRAM
ESSAY TEST

(60 Minutes)

SOCIAL SECURITY NUMBER

Langston, R.

Using your pen, write your social security number in the boxes at the top of the page.

Choose one of the following; put an "X" in the box to indicate your choice.

Essay Topic 185:

"In spite of advances in scientific knowledge, people are still superstitious." Agree or disagree.

Essay Topic 511:

What situations are most stressful for you? Discuss. ✓

Begin your essay on the first lined page. You may use the space below for an outline or notes.
(Remember to use a pen to write your essay. Essays written in pencil will not be graded.)

READING ← LEARNING DISABILITY
        ← FIRST GRADE
        ← READING GROUP
WRITING
ENGLISH   SPELL BY PHOENIX, PHONICS
WRITING ← LITTLE A

ENG ← ONE WORD - LITTLE A NO ENGLISH
    ← ONE WORD AT A TIME
    ← READING

112

Begin writing on this page.   I FIND IT HARD TO DO SOMETHING, I DO NOT KNOW HOW TO DO

THERE ARE MANY SITUATIONS THAT CAN CAUSE STRESS IN A STUDENTS LIFE. FOR ME, READING, WRITING AND ENGLISH ARE THE MOST STRESSFUL ~~FOR SEVERAL REASONS~~ SITUATIONS TO BE IN FOR SEVERAL REASONS. FIRST OF ALL, READING ~~CAN BE VERY HARD IF NOONE EVER TOUGHT~~ IS VERY ^STRESSFUL ~~HARD~~ BECAUSE I WAS NEVER ~~TAUGHT~~ ^TAUGHT HOW TO DO IT. ALSO, ~~WRITING IS THEREF~~ ALSO, WRITING IS STRESSFUL BECAUSE ~~I~~ SPELL THE WAY I READ. ~~FINAL~~ LAST, ENGLISH IS ^THE MOST STRESSFUL BECAUSE IT IS THE ART OF READING AND WRITING.

HOW CAN SOMETHING AS NATURAL AS READING BE ~~HARD~~ STRESSFUL? ~~THE FIRST~~ MY FIRST RUN IN WITH STRESS WAS IN THE FIRST GRADE. MY TEACHER WROTE TWENTY-SIX SYMBOLS ON THE BOARD. THEN SHE REARRANGED THEM ~~INTO~~ HER ^INSTRUCTIONS ~~INSTRUCTIONS~~ AND SAID DO IT! I LOOKED AT ~~THESE~~ ^THE SYMBOLS ON THE BOARD ~~SYMBOLS~~ AND DID WHAT I THOUGHT I SHOULD DO. ~~;~~ I HID IN THE BACK OF THE ROOM EVERYDAY ^FOR THE DAY. WHEN SHE ASKED US TO TURN IN ^AND OUR WORK. ~~WHEN I~~ ^PASSED OUT OF THE FIRST GRADE ~~AND~~ ^AND KNEW ^ONLY ONE SYMBOL ON THE BOARD, THE LETTER "A". I SUCCESSFULY AVOIDED READING UNTIL THE ~~FITH~~ FIFTH GRADE. IN THE FIFTH GRADE MY MOTHER REALIZED I HAD A LEARNING DISABILITY. MY MOTHER FOUND ME HELP IN READING, BUT NOW I HAD TO LEARN TO WRITE.

^LEARNED TO
I ~~WRITE~~ THE WAY EVERY OTHER PERSON ^LEARNS TO WRITE ~~WRITES~~. THE ONLY PROBLEM IS ~~I~~ DO NOT READ LIKE EVERY OTHER PERSON READS. I THOUGHT WRITING WAS EASY UNTIL I LEARNED THAT PHONICS AND SPELLING ARE TWO DIFFERENT WORDS. I LEARNED TO READ BY PHONICS; I SPELL BY PHONICS ^AND ~~AND~~ I SPELL EVERYTHING WRONG. ~~A~~ I HAVE A LOT OF ~~TRABLE~~ ^TROUBLE BELIEVING THAT INTELLIGENCE ~~WAS~~ ^IS NOT SPELLED

For the Children

"INTELLA GENS". I FOUND A WAY TO GET THROUH MY HIGH SCHOOL WRITING DAYS BUT NOT COLLEGE. STRESS IN STRESSFUL SITUATIONS IN COLLEGE ARE CAUSED BY ENGLISH CLASS.

HOW CAN SOMEONE SCREW UP ENGLISH? WHEN EVERY GRADE FROM FIRST THROUGH TWELTH TEACHE ENGLISH. WELL, IT WAS EASY FOR ME. WHEN THE SCHOOL FOUND OUT I HAD A LEARNING DISABILITY THEY DID A BRILLIANT THING. THE SCHOOL SYSTEM TOOK ME OUT OF MY ENGLISH CLASSES EVERY YEAR UNTIL COLLEGE AND TAUGHT ME TO READ. I FOUND MYSELF IN A COLLEGE 101 ENGLISH CLASS AND DIDN'T KNOW WHAT A NOUN WAS. ENGLISH BECAME VERY STRESSFUL TO ME. I HAD TO KNOW IF THIS DOES THAT, THEN THIS DOES THIS AND I DON'T NOT PASS. ENGLISH HAS BEEN A BIG STRUGGLE AND MAJOR STRESS POINT IN MY LIFE.

~~READING IS VERY~~
NOT EVERY PERSON HAS STRESS BECAUSE OF READING, WRITING AND ENGLISH. READING GIVES ME STRESS BECAUSE I WAS NOT TAUGHT HOW TO READ UNTIL THE FIFTH GRADE AND I STILL READ ON A FIFTH GRADE LEVEL. ALSO, WRITING GIVES ME STRESS MY GREAT READING ABILITIES LEAD TO GREAT WRITING DISASTERS DISASTERS THANKS TO PHONICS. THE LAST OF MY STRESS SITUATIONS HAS BEEN ENGLISH. THE BULK OF MY STRESS SITUATIONS HAVE COME FROM ENGLISH. ENGLISH IS THE ART OF READING AND WRITING, AN ART I HOPE TO SOMEDAY MASTER.

The Biggest Mountain

Testing once again became my friend when a seemingly impossible obstacle loomed between me and getting a college degree. I have already told part of this story, but it has a special lesson about testing. You may remember that West Georgia College said I could not get the liberal arts degree for which I had already worked for six years unless I passed two semesters of a foreign language. Given my difficulties with English, I had no doubt that it was out of my learning scope to master a second language. With this knowledge, I revved up my "blue-collar approach" to getting the accommodations I needed.

In my haste to get this problem resolved, I went directly to the Vice President of West Georgia College with my request. He could see how upset I was that this was blocking my way to a college degree. In fact, I had tears in my eyes as I explained my situation and could tell that he empathized with me. However, he said that he could not allow me to substitute other courses for the foreign language. I immediately realized that I had approached my obstacle the wrong way. I learned that it is not always appropriate or effective to start at the top of the educational chain in search of accommodations.

As usual, Dr. Ann Phillips counseled me on the right way to go about my task. First, we needed proof that I was unable to learn a foreign language. Dr. Phillips referred me to The Resource Educational Center, testing by Richard Kaplan, M. Ed., Sp. Ed. The goal of this test was "to determine if Rob has a learning disability in the area of language abstract reasoning. This cognitive processing area is responsible for understanding the analytical skills needed to synthesize linguistic thinking."

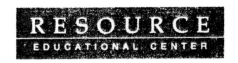

Name: Rob Langston
Age: 23
Birthdate: 11-26-67
Date of Examination: 10-9-91 and 10-11-91

Reason for evaluation:

Rob has had a history of educational problems. Specifically, he expressed that his reading and spelling are very poor. During the intake session Rob expressed classic dyslexic symptoms; such as reversing symbols, slow reading and minimal comprehension. He has worked and struggled to maintain an average grade point status. On his own, during the six years of college to date, Rob has practiced reading in hopes of increasing his skill. This effort has been of benefit and demonstrates his desire and commitment to help himself. Although he emotionally is hurt by academic obstacles, Rob has attempted most collegic demands independent of special assistance for which he is qualified.

Rob has established himself as a motivational speaker specializing in overcoming obstacles. This forum is a constructive outlet for his own frustrations. However, he must overcome his foreign language requirements for him to continue to believe in himself. This academic requirement appears to be one that he can't cope with independently.

Test Administered:

Woodcock-Johnson - Revised
Test of Cognitive Ability:

	Age	Grade
Memory for Names	3-6	K.0
Visual Matching	10-11	5.4
Incomplete Words	7-6	2.4
Visual Closure	24	16.9
Analysis-Synthesis	31	16.9
Visual-Auditory Learning	25	16.9
Memory for Words	17-10	11.9
Cross-Out	25	16.9

Rob Langston
Examination Dates: 10-9-91 and 10-11-91
Page 2

Test of Achievement:	Age	Grade
Sound Blending	26	16.8
Oral Vocabulary	16-10	11.2
Delayed Recall	15-7	9.7
Number Reversed	8-8	3.4
Spatial Relations	30	16.4
Word Identification	12-0	6.7
Passage Comprehension	16-6	11.0
Dictation	9-9	4.3
Writing Samples	17-7	11.7
Word Attack	9-4	4.1
Proofing	10-1	4.6
Punctuation	8-11	3.3
Spelling	9-9	4.3
Usage	12-10	7.4

Test Interpretation:

This psycho-educational battery specifically was administered to determine if Rob has a learning disability in the area of language abstract reasoning. This cognitive processing area is responsible for understanding the analytical skills needed to synthesize linguistic thinking. In addition to this cognitive process, Rob's visual and auditory perceptions were evaluated to determine if blocks may be occurring between his eyes or ears and intellectual ability.

In reviewing Rob's evaluation, it is evident that there is a significant amount of intra-test scatter. This inconsistency demonstrates that Rob will find certain academic challenges to be mastered easily and appropriately; and others to be extremely difficult, if not impossible to master. This range of functioning is inconsistent with his intellectual ability.

Specific psycho-educational weaknesses assessed include his inability to retain information that does not have logical meaning. This lag accounts for his very slow process in learning how to read. As a self-taught reader, he needs an abundance of repetition in order for him to remember the written word. This was only accomplished after he slowly developed a basic working sight vocabulary. From this development and maturity, Rob started to read material which was logical and sequential. This method allowed him to use his comprehension skills as the key for the next word in the sentence. Over the last few years Rob has now learned to read, however, as indicated on this assessment, he is only functioning at year-end six grade level in sight vocabulary. His passage comprehension skill is substantially above that placement.

This lack of memory or the ability to store details was cognitively assessed when comparing the memory for names and the visual-auditory learning sub-tests. The same perceptual skills are used, however, the latter sub-test is logically based. This substantial weakness creates numerous academic problems other than the reading example cited above. Rob will have difficulty remembering the multiplication tables, mathematical formulas, sequence of operations or processes, spelling, names, dates and learning foreign languages.

This battery of testing also assessed Rob to have visual receptive difficulties when stimuli is similar. It appears that visual information is not perceived in the correct order. This simple operation, but important process, contributes to Rob's academic slowness, and weak academic skill listed previously. It is important to note, that when visual stimuli was presented that was not similar, he did much better. This indicates that Rob will not have a problem visualizing non-language stimuli.

Auditorally, Rob demonstrated similar inconsistencies. When information was presented logically, his memory was much better than when presented with little meaning. This indicates that he has poor auditory concentration or long term memory. This lag was also demonstrated on the Delayed Recall sub-test.

It should be noted that Rob's ability to analyze and synthesize concepts is very good. This important strength has been the foundation of most of his learning.

The Test of Achievement assessed all language-based skills to be weak. These problems are the symptoms of the weak cognitive process discussed above.

Rob's weak academic foundation prevents him from identifying mis-spelled words or grammatical errors, and limited strategy base to read complicated material on his intellectual level.

Given the psycho-educational problems and his lack of English language technical skills, Rob will not be able to learn a foreign language which is taught in a classroom. His desire to learn and to be normal is evident. But his learning disability will prevent him from being successful.

Rob needs to concentrate on his native language skills, as well as to develop his weak cognitive skills so he can function on his intellectual level. This should be of priority so that he can emotionally heal and achieve success on what level he chooses.

118

Their report said, "He must overcome his foreign language requirements for him to believe in himself." I could not have said it better. But could I learn a foreign language, given my learning disabilities? The test showed that I had a "significant amount of intra-test scatter." It went on to say, "This inconsistency demonstrates that Rob will find certain academic challenges to be mastered easily and appropriately; and others to be extremely difficult, if not impossible to master. This range of functioning is inconsistent with his intellectual ability."

In this comprehensive analysis, my learning disability was fully explained. They looked for and found the variances, the difference between scores for a variety of skills that were indicative of learning disabilities. The test showed that I was extremely deficient in some ways and extremely proficient in others. At twenty-three years old, I scored on a kindergarten level on "memory for names," and on a thirty-year-old level for "special relations." This was the proof that I had a learning disability.

The bottom line was, "Given the psycho-educational problems and his lack of English language technical skills, Rob will not be able to learn a foreign language, which is taught in a classroom."

I now had the documentation I needed to go to the Dean of my department and request substitutions for the foreign language requirement. I did and he said, "Yes." He gave his approval for the substitution.

The Choice is Yours

Testing can be your friend or your enemy. If you prepare yourself mentally for the down side of testing, you can survive with your self-esteem intact. Again, keep your focus on what you hope to accomplish through the testing. Remember, that testing builds that all-important paper trail that educators love. Your educational history follows you through college and gives you the credentials to receive accommodations.

Remember that tests results do not indicate who you are or what you know. Testing reports are not an accurate representation of a student's ability to succeed in life. Outlook, imagination, and motivation are the keys to success. Accept testing, use it for your benefit, and then forget it.

CHAPTER 8

The Future of Education is Special Education

A few years ago, I had a wake-up call.

I had already been talking to people for years about learning disabilities. I knew the message I wanted to deliver from my own experience, and both teachers and students seemed to be inspired by what I said. But after what happened that day, I gained a much larger perspective.

Rob, They Want You at the Prison!

One hot July morning, my secretary called into my office, "Rob, I have Fulton County Prison on the phone. They want to talk to you!"

"Tell them I'm not here," I yelled.

She laughed and called in to me, "No, they want you to come down and do your program."

Reluctantly, I picked up the phone and said in my most professional voice, "Hello, this is Rob Langston."

The person on the other end of the line explained that she would like for me to give my motivational program to the prisoners.

"No!" I said without hesitation, "I worked very hard to stay out of your prison when I was younger and I have no desire whatsoever to go down there for any reason." At this point, it was easy to forget that my goal was to help others.

"Well, when The Kroger Company calls, you do it." I could tell by her voice that she knew she had me. Kroger was the corporate sponsor through whom I spoke to more than 20,000 students each year. I wasn't about to bite the hand that fed me, and she knew it. This was a command performance. I wrote the date down on my calendar and promptly dismissed the talk from my mind.

Prison day finally arrived. Most speakers begin preparing for a talk from the moment they wake up, and I am no different. I went through my normal wake-up routine, and put on my best, casual clothes. I looked in the mirror, squared my shoulders, lifted my chin, put a smile on my face, and said aloud, "Whoever needs you will hear you today."

As I drove down I-20 to Fulton County Prison, I continued the positive self-talk and reviewed in my mind what I wanted to say. My enthusiasm continued to build and I was excited at the chance to share my story.

But when I got within about five miles of the facility, I saw it for the first time. It is a ten-story building, and from a distance I could see tiny windows on each floor. As I got closer, I realized that the windows were actually just little gun slats. As I drove closer and closer, and finally turned into the parking lot, the building looked more and more ominous. I started thinking, 'Rob, what have you gotten yourself into?' I looked up at the huge gray stone building, and my positive self-talk was all but forgotten.

I got out of the car and started walking slowly toward the building with my cinder blocks and wooden boards for my "overcoming obstacles" demonstration tucked under my arms. With more than a little trepidation, I walked up to the door and said, "I'm Rob Langston and I am here to do a program."

Bring in The Prisoners!

They let me in, and then quickly grabbed the metal detectors and scanned my entire body. They took my driver's license; checked it to make sure I was who I said I was and put a badge around my neck so I could get back out. At this point, I was starting to shake.

The woman who had invited me came in and shook my hand. "Follow me," she said.

"Yes ma'am, whatever you say," I answered quickly. She unlocked the first set of iron doors. We walked through, and I jumped as the doors clanged shut behind me. I'm here to tell you those doors sound exactly like they do in the movies. They clang shut, they are LOUD, and we had to go through two more of them. By the time that third door banged behind me, my nerves were shot. Panic had set in. Perspiration beaded my forehead and tightness gripped my chest. My only thought was 'I have to get out of here and quick!' But there was no turning back.

Finally, we got to the cellblock and the lady stood me right in the center. I looked up and saw two tiers of cells. That was all these prisoners were going to see for the next five years of their lives. On the way in, I asked the lady about the group I would be addressing. She said, "Everybody here today has a minimum sentence of five years. You will be speaking to drug dealers, murderers, rapist and thieves. The worst of the worst."

My first thought was, "This is not a group I want to disappoint."

Suddenly I heard this big booming voice say, "Bring in the prisoners!"

I huddled over to the side while the lady gave me a flowery introduction. When she was finished, I turned around to face my audience. Nothing came out of my mouth. Not because I did not know what to say, but because what I saw shocked me. Staring back at me was a sea of despairing, disinterested faces; they were young. They were all about thirteen to sixteen years old. I turned to the lady.

"What are they doing here?" I asked her.

"Nobody told you?" She asked.

"Told me what?"

"We brought you here to speak to juveniles," she said. "All these kids were tried as adults. The oldest person in the room is sixteen." These were the faces with no hope. I was shocked and heartsick. 'How could this be? What had gone wrong?' Then I had a shocking realization. Only by the grace of God and the help of a stubborn, strong-willed mother had I escaped being one of these young faces before me.

"But why me?" I asked. "I speak in the educational system on learning disabilities and overcoming obstacles. Why am I here?"

"That is exactly why you are here," she said. "We believe that 80% of the Georgia penal system is made up of either learning disabled people or illiterates." I was astounded, "You are telling me that if they don't make it in school, in our institutions of higher education, then they are ending up in institutions of incarceration?"

"That is it exactly," she said.

What I Learned that Day

I needed to convince myself that giving this talk was a good idea, and quickly. I remembered that these young people needed to hear my message. Maybe my story about overcoming obstacles to find success, happiness and self-worth would change something for them.

I imagined they were looking at me and thinking that I had lived a charmed life, but I knew that it was the difficulties that had molded my character. I might be a middle class kid from the suburbs, but my life had not been easy. Life is difficult when your brain does not function in the same way as others, which means that you cannot learn the way other people learn. Some of the prisoners sitting in front of me had probably had the same problem. School had been hard for me, and it had probably been hard or impossible for most of them.

With these thoughts in mind, I relaxed and spoke to the young inmates about my experience in school, what I had learned, and the principles I had applied to succeed. They listened as I gave my talk about overcoming obstacles to achieve success. I have no way of knowing if I touched a cord in any of them, but it was obvious to me that they were not all as tough as they pretended to be. They were kids with broken hearts and destroyed dreams. They were young people whom the educational system most likely had failed.

Helping People Early

After that talk at the prison, I wanted to learn more about the possibility that many people are in prison because they failed in school. Donn O. Smith is Program Development Consultant for Special Education and

Juvenile Services for the State of Georgia Department of Corrections. He gave me a lot of information that reinforced my conviction that if we can catch students with learning disabilities early and give them what they need to learn, they can become productive members of society. If we can do that, we not only save individual lives, but we create a society in which everyone contributes, rather than takes from the whole.

Donn shared with me the results from observing Georgia prisoners who were given the WRAT (Wide Range Achievement Test, which measures reading, writing and math levels) and an IQ test that was culturally unbiased when they entered prison.[13] Of the more than 6,000 inmates who were tested, 23% read at a 3rd grade or lower level and more than 60% read at a 5.9 or lower grade level. A reading level below the 6th grade indicates functional illiteracy. If this study is representative of the whole prison population, then well over half of all prisoners are functionally illiterate. Although we have no facts concerning the cause of the prisoners' illiteracy, my suspicion is that many of them have learning disabilities.[14]

As I listened to Donn, I realized that although he was talking about people who were incarcerated in Georgia, much of what he said applied to people on welfare, to people on the streets, and to people who were just getting by and not living very happy or productive lives.

The Bigger Picture

The Georgia prison system is just a microcosm of a problem, which exists on a much larger scale. Millions of people are involved in this scenario. Experts disagree on the number of people in the United States who have learning disabilities and particularly on the number of people with dyslexia, but the estimate range is from 5% to 25% of the population. If we use a median figure of 10%, at least 25 million people are affected.

People with learning disabilities who have not had their needs met by the educational system do not always wind up in prison. Sometimes they go on welfare, or have to struggle just to get by. The presence of undiagnosed learning disabilities in a high percentage of low-income people greatly impedes governmental efforts to effectively provide a wide range of services aimed at alleviating poverty in the population.

Approximately 48% of those out of work or unemployed have learning disabilities and 25%-35% of welfare recipients have learning disabilities. A report titled "Functional Impairments of AFDC Clients," from the J.S. Department of Health and Human Services states that many adults with learning disabilities were never identified as being learning disabled when they were in school, and so they never received any special education. Most were not even aware that they had problems.

People with learning disabilities may have new opportunities as a result of the current labor shortage. The Georgia Department of Labor has expressed an interest in developing employees who can function at their "full capacity." Through testing, they hope to identify certain learning problems and then match peoples' skills with specific jobs.

We all pay for education, incarceration and welfare. We can put our money into educating people in ways that work, or we can pay for their incarceration and welfare. It's just that simple. Education makes for a better quality of life, and it is a lot less expensive.

What I Believe

I believe that the future of education is special education, which is based on discovering people's individual learning styles and using their strengths instead of beating up on their weaknesses.

Every child who can learn has the right to learn and should be given the chance to learn. Helping people early can make everybody more productive and fulfilled. We need to find out what problems people have with learning, and what each person's individual learning needs are, and then give them what they need in order to learn. That will transform our society. It will make us all givers rather than takers. It will free up the time, energy and money we now spend on punishing people or giving them welfare and provide for more productive activities. We will have more teachers, more facilities and more capacity to keep people out of trouble.

If children are not making it in the institutions of education, they are not making it. When we don't give students what they need to learn, we become a society that is merely warehousing human beings. Some of these people are very bright. All they need is a break. What can we do? Early intervention, which keeps children in school helps steer them away from trouble and gets them into the work force as productive citizens. Donn says, "If we can give some kids successes in school, maybe we can overcome bad home situations."

My message to young people with learning disabilities is that the prison scenario does not have to be their scenario. People with learning disabilities can become able and successful in lawful, productive ways. I am living proof of that.

Commitment and determination are crucial, but the key element in whether children succeed or fail is self-esteem.

Self-Esteem: The Key Ingredient

I tell people that reading, writing, and arithmetic are not as important as self-esteem. Many educators are stunned, and don't believe me when I say this. After all, their livelihood depends on teaching reading, writing and arithmetic and on using the three "Rs" to teach other subjects.

I got through most of my life without reading, writing and arithmetic, but I never would have made it without self-esteem. My mother was told when I was in elementary school that I would never go to college. They said I simply did not have the higher faculties to make it. If she had believed them, and if I had just given up, I very likely would have been in the audience at Fulton County Prison instead of giving the talk.

Learning disabilities have always been with us, but they have been hidden behind a veil of embarrassment and disgrace. Both my father and my paternal grandfather had dyslexia. In their generations, and even to some extent in mine, learning disabilities have been cloaked in mystery and non-acceptance. Students with learning disabilities were called "dumb" or "disturbed." They did their best to tough it out. They suffered inwardly, and worked hard to be considered "normal" members of society.

It was very difficult to have high self-esteem under those conditions. I often think of the pain my grandfather must have felt as a child and young adult as he watched his four brilliant siblings excel in school and get advanced degrees while he struggled to learn. He dropped out of high school but after he married, he took and passed the GED test to get a high school diploma and become an enormous success in business. He went on to be President and owner of Great Dane Trailer Sales.

Today, we know more about learning disabilities and have seen that even very bright people can have trouble learning. People are likely to be more understanding, but the bottom line is that it is up to each one of us to maintain and nurture our own self-esteem, then do the same for those we love who are learning disabled.

Therefore, the most important lessons are to give students what they need in order to learn in their own way and to foster their self-esteem. I had the benefit of both these keys to success. Long before my teachers recognized that I was smart, my family knew it. Over the years, many people have remarked to me that my mom must have known a lot about learning disabilities when I was growing up. The truth is, she knew nothing about them during my early childhood. What she did know was that she had a smart child at home who was failing in school. She observed that I had a large vocabulary, used complex words correctly, and was accepted as an equal by smart children. So she and my father based all of their decisions about my education on the premise that I was smart, but that I learned differently from other kids. She got me what I needed in order to learn, and she never let my self-esteem suffer.

Lifelong Learners

My mission is to help all learning-disabled students find a way to survive the school system with their self-esteem intact, so that they become lifelong learners. I want them to find their strengths and passions. I want them to pursue learning with joy. To be a lifelong learner is an incomparable gift, that no one can give to you. You have to take a stand in favor of education. Teachers and parents have to provide support and encouragement. That is why teachers and parents of learning disabled students do life-or-death work. I know because I was one of their students.

I believe that everybody wants to learn. Nobody wants to be considered stupid. You can misbehave in school and be cool, but you can not be dumb and be cool. Even first graders know that. It is just a matter of creating an environment in which everybody can learn. That is the change we need to make in the educational system today.

The first step in becoming a lifelong learner, or in helping children become lifelong learners, is to recognize that people who have trouble learning are not dumb. Children talk to themselves every waking moment. They give themselves messages all the time. It is important that those messages are positive. Children need to know that they are smart, even if they have a learning disorder. This will keep their self-esteem high enough that they can go after and accept the support they need to learn in their own way. When they master that art of learning in their own way and in their own style, they naturally become lifelong learners.

I remember one little kid who came up to me after a program and said, "Rob, I love what you said, but I can't wait until I get out of school so I can stop learning."

I said to him, "Did you hear what you just said?"

"Yes, I want to get out of school so I can quit learning," he said.

"What is it about learning that hurts you?" I asked him.

"The tests," he said.

It is very important for this young man to recognize and change how he is talking to himself, because he is listening to his own reflections. With the messages he is giving himself now, he will quit learning after graduation, if he makes it to graduation. The tragedy is that he does not really want to quit learning. What he really wants is to stop hurting, and that means being tested differently, in a way that meets his needs, so he will not feel dumb. When and if that happens, he will be free to be a lifelong learner.

Everything I know about learning disabilities, I know from my own personal experience. My story illustrates both the dangers and the possibilities of being learning disabled. What I learned from being dyslexic enabled me to succeed in every area of my life. I am not special. Armed with information, self-esteem, and a desire to be a lifelong learner, everyone can do what I did.

Part 4: Thriving and Succeeding

CHAPTER 9

Principles for Thriving with Your Disability

In the preceding chapters, I have talked about my vision, my story and some of the tools that learning disabled people can use to survive and thrive in the educational system and in life. In this chapter, I want to tie it all together and give you a set of principles that you can use to be an able person and a lifelong learner.

Here are the principles that helped me succeed despite my learning disability:

If you have a problem, tell someone and get help. Before I finally told my mother, "I can't write what I know," my life was filled with fear. I had to figure out how to lie, hide and cheat each day so that no one would find out how poorly I read. I do not know what would have happened to me if I had kept on that path. I surely would not have gotten the help I needed.

Once I had shared my secret with Mom, she became my advocate. She started speaking to teachers on my behalf. She researched and explored learning disabilities and searched for an answer to what was wrong with me. She sent me to Dr. Levinson and other experts. She made sure I had what I needed in order to learn in school each day. Without that help, it is unlikely I would have completed my schooling.

My mother had an unspoken agreement of support with me. I never doubted that she would stay by my side no matter what the situation. My part of the agreement was that I would tell her the truth. She would say, "Do not let the phone ring with someone reporting something about you that you have not told me. You had better tell me first." Of course, it was easy to tell the truth knowing that she would be non-judgmental and supportive. My mother now says that she knew that if she wavered from her rule of standing by my side even one time, she would lose my trust.

When I told my friends about my disability the day we were all gathered around the new video game, I opened up even more possibilities. Instead of hiding my disability from the people I hung out with every day, I could relax and be who I was. I knew that they accepted me even with my disability. That acceptance contributed enormously to my self-esteem and to my enjoyment of life.

It takes courage to talk about a disability, especially at first. The rewards far outweigh the discomfort and the truth is, you can not go forward until you share your problem and let people know.

Focus on the solution.

If you have a problem, no matter how thick and hard it is, concentrate on the solution. Do not get caught up in the problem and let it drag you down.

Remember the demonstration I do at the end of my talks? I set two inch-thick boards on cinder blocks and break them with my hand.

I use two boards because there are two sets of problems we have to worry about in life. The first set is society's problems such as drugs, alcohol, poverty, disease, and violence. You may not want to deal with these things, but they are with us and most of us have to confront them on some level. The second set of problems is personal. Many of my personal problems had to do with my learning disability.

When you run into these problems, they are going to try and stop you. Do not let them. The way I break through those boards is not to concentrate on the boards. If I did that, I would break my hand and wrist every time. I concentrate on the floor beneath the boards. That is the solution. That is where I want my hand to go. It is going to have to go through the boards to get there. When you concentrate on the solution, you pass right through the problem.

I have practiced this technique over time both with the boards and in life. I have developed the habit of focusing on the solution rather than dwelling on the problem. My mind now goes immediately to the positive outcome that I want. The solution may be to ask a particular person for help. Rarely do I encounter someone who is not willing to help. In fact, when they are not willing to help, I feel sorry for them. They have not learned the valuable lesson I have learned from being learning disabled. We are here to share our talents and to help others. I do not let these people affect my mood, my confidence, or my self-image. I do not let them determine who I am, how I feel, or the success I achieve.

Learning disabilities are only learning disabilities. They do not mean you are not smart.

You can struggle in school and still be very intelligent. Many learning disabilities are physical disabilities, not mental ones.

I remember so clearly the relief I felt after being given an IQ test that did not depend on my ability to read and write. When I discovered through that test that I actually had above average intelligence, a whole new world opened up to me. I could relax and I could succeed.

Dr. Howard Gardner of Harvard University has a new view of intelligence and of learning. He believes that our current tests often fail to identify true intelligence. He says that the standard IQ test basically measures two notions, "intelligence" and "ability," with words and with numbers. Children who score high on the test will be successful in school as it is being taught today. The reason is, that our school system teaches to these intelligences, Linguistic and Logical-Mathematical Intelligence. But it does not mean that they are fundamentally more intelligent than other people.

In *Frames of Mind,* Dr. Gardner relates his theory of multiple intelligence. These include Linguistic Intelligence, Logical-Mathematical Intelligence, Visual-Spatial Intelligence, Musical Intelligence, Bodily-Kinesthetic Intelligence, Interpersonal (social) Intelligence, and Naturalist Intelligence. Our school system does not take this range of intelligence into consideration when it judges who is "smart." It rewards only those students who are proficient in words and numbers.[15]

What about the concert pianist who has difficulty verbalizing her thoughts? Or the real estate Million Dollar Round Table member who cannot write? Consider the person who speaks to and motivates 20,000 children, parents, and teachers a year to love themselves and develop their talents. This is a creative problem solver who displays artistic talent but spent most of his life without being able to read, write or do math. Is he less valuable than the college professor? I do not think he is less, he has wisdom to share. I am that person.

Being called "dumb" and "stupid," or some other negative term has scarred many people with learning disabilities. As we come to know more about learning disabilities, this happens with less frequency, but it is crucial that students do not buy into this negative labeling.

Find your own learning style and use it. As I have said, I believe the future of education is special education. In an ideal situation, each special education student has a group of people sitting around a table discussing his needs. Anyone with a vest interest in the child's future, which includes parents, family, teachers, etc. is sitting around that table talking about what that student needs in order to learn and how they can get those needs met for him.

Why is this limited to special education students? I believe that is what it will take to get all of our children a good education. If we simply address each student's individual learning style early, when they first start school, we will not have to label people "learning disabled." Each person will simply have his or her particular style of learning. One day perhaps the educational system will accommodate all those individual needs.

The new consciousness in education should be: We all learn differently. That is okay. Everyone should have his or her needs met in the classroom. Until that time, take control of your own education. Find out about your learning styles and use the information in this book to get the accommodations you need.

Be your own advocate.

Some of us are blessed with parents and teachers who are our advocates when we are young. Although at some point, we all have to become our own advocate. We need to know our needs and go about getting them met in whatever way works best for us. Before anyone was accommodating for learning disabilities at West Georgia College, I used my "blue collar approach." In a courteous, respectful but determined way, I asked people for what I needed. If I did not get my needs met with that person, I asked someone else until I got what I was asking for.

I learned to be an advocate for myself from watching my mother as my advocate. Now I am an advocate for millions. When an advocate goes after an accommodation, there is action and results.

Keep your self-esteem intact.

Check your attitude. Do you have a positive attitude for education, for success, and for yourself? Keep your self-esteem high at any cost.

My attitude about self-esteem also came from watching my mother. Every year, she dragged me kicking and screaming to parent-teacher conferences. I hated them, but I paid attention when my parents talked to my teachers. My mother began these conversations with, "Rob is extremely intelligent, but he needs..." Then she would go on to tell the teacher whatever it was I needed. At the close of the conference, my mother would reiterate, "Rob is extremely intelligent." Those statements reinforced that I was intelligent! She was doing whatever it took to keep my self-esteem intact, despite some rough going in the early years.

When students fail in the education system, they often lose respect for themselves. Their low self-esteem is actually created and perpetuated by the educational system. In turn, low self-esteem creates and perpetuates a society of angry young people who are more likely to turn to violence and crime.

The solution is to educate all our children and make them feel that they are worthwhile members of society. Every young person should emerge from our educational system as a lifelong learner and a contributing member of society. Education is not a place but a state of mind. Lifelong learners will succeed in spit of disabilities.

Ask for what you want and do not be afraid of the bureaucracy.

Remember the system is more flexible than you think. Especially if you have established precedents and are willing to be persistent and go the distance. You can get what you want and need.

Also remember the other side of this coin. Neither the government nor the educational system will change unless you demand it. They are essentially static institutions that will bend and change under pressure. You have to be an advocate and by being one you can get results, if you stick with it.

For instance, can you pick your teachers in elementary school? You bet you can. You can certainly avoid teachers you do not want. Schools hate for me to tell parents that, but I do. I learned by watching my mother. This story is about my mother and my sister Natalie, who does not have a learning disorder.

My mother took Natalie to school on the first day of

first grade and there was a substitute teacher. Mom was not pleased. She was told that Natalie's teacher was recovering from back surgery and would be back in a few days. A week later, there was a new substitute teacher. Again Mom was assured the classroom teacher would be back in just a day or two. When the third substitute teacher arrived, Mom was through waiting. She walked into the principal's office. He had been dealing with Mom for six years, so he took one look at her and said, "do whatever you want, Martha! I do not even want to hear about it."

Mom took Natalie down to the teacher that my brother and I had in first grade. She introduced Natalie to Mrs. Bailey. After introductions, Mom sat Natalie down and said, "This is your new class." She walked out and the problem was solved. It is simple if you take on my mother's motto: "If my children do not survive in education today, they do not survive."

The key is to get involved. Someone once asked me if I could only say one thing to parents, what would it be? I answered this way, "If you can do one thing as a parent, get involved in your child's education." Education is a two-way street. The educational system must take responsibility for providing the teachers and the tools for learning. Parents and students must take responsibility for wanting to learn. In all my school years, I brought to the table an eagerness and enthusiasm to learn. People responded to this and helped me get what I needed.

Until our educational system is able to provide learning disabled students with what they need as a matter of course, it is up to parents to develop the "attitude for education" as my mother did. It is the attitude that your child will be educated no matter what it takes.

Today, parents of learning disabled students have an ally in an unlikely place, the government. In 1997, Congress passed the re-authorization of IDEA (Individuals with Disabilities Education Act), which states, "the educational needs of more than 8 million children with disabilities in the United States are not being met." IDEA continues, "It is in the national interest that the federal government assist state and local efforts to provide programs to meet the educational needs of children with disabilities in order to assure equal protection of the law."

The Federation of Families for Children's Mental Health states, that IDEA guarantees children with disabilities a free, appropriate, public education in the least restrictive environment. The Federation goes on to explain that "the state must provide all members of a class of individuals (students) the same opportunity to participate and benefit." The law does not spell out the type of service each child must receive, but decrees that each child will receive services appropriate to their circumstances.[16]

As a result of IDEA, parents have the right and responsibility to direct their children's education. We have seen that if a parent can show in the IEP (Individualized Education Plan) Group that a child learns better under certain conditions, then the school must meet that need.

The Individuals with Disabilities Education Act amendments of 1999, provides accommodations for these conditions. The drawback is that the parents and teachers do not regularly recognize or acknowledge a child's disability in the early years. In my case I lied, cheated, hid and memorized so that the teachers were not aware of the extent of my disability until the 5th grade. My family did recognize my disabilities.[17]

The ball is now in the parents' court. It is up to them to take the initiative to identify their children's learning problems, and parents are actually the ones best equipped to determine their children's learning styles. Parents can diagnose the child's learning styles by talking to him, watching him play, watching what motivates and excites him. Trial and error also plays a part. Ask the child to draw a picture depicting a story in the history book. Sing or rhyme her lessons. Read to him and let him become an actor, dramatizing his reading or history lessons. To which learning style does he respond to best? Is math a mystery until objects are used to solve math problems? Read about learning disabilities and learning styles. Educate yourself and become the resident expert in your household.

Parents who work with their children know how they learn. Here are two examples of this fact at work.

When I was in high school, we had final exams at the end of each semester. There were two two-hour exams a day with three hours in between. We were not allowed to leave campus between the two exams. Mom would come and sign me out so we could go study for the second exam. We would sit at McDonald's and make up silly sentences for list of things I needed to know. I could remember the silly sentences and with them the information.

My sister dated a guy in college with a learning disability. She called my mother and explained that the silly sentence method was not working for her friend. My sister later talked to his mother and found out that he had a different learning style. His mother knew how he could learn, just as my mother had known about me.

Work with people, not against them.

My mother stressed that no matter how firm my demands, I should also be polite. When parents start advocating for their children, they often start seeing teachers as the enemy. Nothing could be farther from the truth. Teachers have a difficult and thankless job. They have my deepest admiration. Because many teachers get bogged down in paperwork and red tape trying to satisfy the school administration and the government, they must sometimes sacrifice their focus on the children's perform-ance to carry out their administrative duties.

To continue in defense of teachers, I have seen par-ents who do not do their share. Teachers tell me that they try to get the parents involved, but parents will not even return telephone calls. This is sad, but the teacher still does not have the right to give up on the child. When the child comes from an unstable home environment, the school system is in a position to provide stability.

In addition to the friction between teachers and par-ents, there is friction between special education teachers and regular education teachers. Teachers and adminis-trators often do not see eye to eye. While all these con-flicts are being played out, education slows down and the children suffer.

Keep the love of life and learning alive.

Many experts now say that the conditions for effective learning include a child-like, supportive, and playful envi-ronment.

Recently, I was speaking to an elementary school parents' group and one mother approached me. Earlier that day I had also spoken to the students at that school. The woman told me that her son had come home to tell her that a "man talked to us at school today."

"Who was he?" she asked.

The child reflected for a moment and then answered, "He was a student." Upon further reflection, he corrected himself, "No, he was like me."

This eight-year-old child felt he had something in common with a thirty-year-old man. I feel the reason is that I am childlike and still have a child's enthusiasm to learn. My feelings are not hurt when people accuse me of being a child. If being a child means that I have a child's joy in play, curiosity to learn, and wonder of discovery, I am delighted.

Many adults walk around without much joy and happiness in their lives because they believe that life is a struggle and that adults should be serious-minded. Perhaps by seeing this in their parents and by being subjected to this attitude in our schools, children lose their love of life and their love of learning. Students can laugh and play their way to success in school. And, adults can have fun as they pursue their life's dreams. A bright smile and a kind word can point one on the path to fulfillment instead of the path to destruction.

Take the fear out of the classroom.

I have told the story of the teacher going around the class asking each child to read a paragraph. I would count the children before me so I could determine what para-

graph I would be asked to read and then frantically practice until it was my turn. Even then, I could not read the
paragraph and was so humiliated that I went home crying.
When I told my mother about this, she talked to the
teacher and arranged that I not be asked to read aloud.

The lesson Mom taught me from this incident was that
it was up to me to "be bigger than adults." This translated
into my speaking up when called on to read and saying,
"My mother said I do not have to read aloud in class." The
teacher then remembered the conference and her agreement with my mother, and I was not called on to read.
Most teachers are overworked, underpaid, and have too
many students. In addition, they are human beings. If they
forget what your needs are, it is up to you to remind them.

Mom not only told me that I did not have to do anything in class that embarrassed me, she gave me the
words to say to the teacher to avoid difficult situations. At
home, she had me practice saying them over and over.
That empowered me to stand up for myself at an early
age, and took the fear out of the classroom for me.

Focus on your strengths.

Learning to focus on my strengths was a large part of
my success. I have good people skills. I care. I speak
well. Even in school, I focused on people and on being of
service, in football (where my strength might have been
psychological rather than physical, but was there
nonetheless), and in the fraternity.

Another way I focused on my strengths was to change
my major from business to fine arts. I first chose a business major because that's what all the men in my family
had done. Successful business men and entrepreneurs

were greatly admired among my family. After careful consideration, I realized that it made more sense for me to focus on a fine arts degree. I love art and have talent in that area. By focusing on these strengths, I was able to draw and paint my way to a college degree. I received many honors and awards along the way as well. Today, am I less respected by the "business degree" men in my family? No! In fact, in 1997 I was listed in the International Who's Who of Entrepreneurs. Not too bad for not having a business degree. The point here is: focus on your strengths because a degree is a degree is a degree.

Which brings me to a point I have not discussed thus far. Money for the arts is slowly drying up in the schools. Many legislators and administrators consider art, music, physical education and dance educational "fluff," and of no real educational value. They do not understand that as they eliminate the arts from school, they are also crushing creative thinking, problem solving, and brain development. Many students who learn differently excel in careers using their creative abilities. A great avenue for expressing themselves and building positive self-esteem is taken away. I would never have known that I was good at art if I had not been able to take art classes in high school.

Keep going.

Learning-disabled people teach themselves to live with adversity and disappointment. Some will not be accepted into college. They should not let this stop the learning. Learning does not end with formal schooling. As a recruiter for the State University of West Georgia, I was asked by the Admissions Department to write a letter of encouragement to a high school student who had not been accepted by the school. The first thing I said to him was "Education is not a place. Education is a state of mind." I encouraged them to investigate other college programs. And even if someone was not accepted the first time, the second time, or even the third time, they should continue trying.

Reference books in the public library list several hundred colleges and universities that have special accommodations for students with learning disabilities. For example, the State University of West Georgia now actively pursues students with disabilities characterized as Physical, Psychological, or Learning Disorders. Dr. Ann Phillips and her staff in the University's Department of Disabled Student Services have developed a booklet that enumerates the many accommodations the university now offers these students.

The accommodations include:

- Student Disability Report
- Time Management Training
- Testing Accommodations
- Student Anchor
- Note Taking Assistance
- Foreign Language Substitution
- Taping Lectures
- Interpreters
- Preferred Seating
- Closed Caption TV
- Readers Assistance

- Hearing Device
- Books on Tape
- Software
- Specialized Advising
- Special Furniture
- Early Bird Registration
- Campus Mobility Training
- Drop/Add
- Early Class Registration
- Modification of Class Activities
- Tutoring
- Assistance Pulling Library Material

A South Georgia school superintendent told me he knew of a learning disabled student who did not pass the high school exit exam for Georgia because of a lack of accommodations. Earlier that year this same student had been accepted by Yale, after receiving the accommodations on their entrance exam pending high school graduation. I strongly believe that if we want something badly enough, we will find a way to get it.

These are the principles you can use if you are learning disabled. In the next chapter, I will present my formula for success for everybody.

CHAPTER 10

A Formula for Success

Success means different things to each of us. To one person, it may mean being the CEO of a global enterprise. To another, it may mean a loving family.

Each of us has a vast, untapped potential that can take us wherever we want to go. My goal is to help you unleash your talents and abilities, although you have to determine what success is to you, create your blueprint, and plan strategies for achieving your goals.

The Path to Success is Paved with Self-esteem

One common denominator of successful people is self-esteem. You have to believe in yourself.

I only started to reach my goals after I developed healthy self-esteem. Coming to this belief in myself was not easy. I had to overcome a background of failure in school. I was often told that my learning disability would limit me in life and that I could not achieve certain goals because of my "handicap." But I learned not to accept what other people thought of me if it did not support my success. I had to retrain my mind to believe that academic success was not the ultimate or only success. I had to accept the fact that I could not read or do math well, although I could be successful. My family was a tremendous help. They always believed I was smart, talented, and special, and they never once wavered from this belief.

Today, I make a rule that what other people think of me is none of my business. Wayne Dyer says, "You have to be independent of the good opinion of others."

For me, the key to developing self-esteem was to embrace and internalize the image of a capable, valuable person. For this, I needed to change my perception of myself. I worked diligently to internalize new beliefs until they became my reality. Some people tell me, "That is easier said than done." I agree. It is difficult to change from a lifetime of negative perceptions to a future of positive perceptions. But it can be done.

The Marines do a great job of this. They have the difficult chore of teaching young men to overcome their fear and charge forward while staring down the barrel of a machine gun. They practice this activity over and over and over again until it becomes an automatic response. They become desensitized to normal fear. Self-esteem works the same way. We must practice success over and over until it is an integral part of our makeup. When success becomes a conditioned response, we automatically reject obstacles, criticism, and others' negativity. Success leaves footprints.

If self-esteem is not internalized on a deep level, we can forget what we know in a heartbeat. On the *Getting What You Really, Really, Really Want* tape, Wayne Dyer tells the story of squeezing an orange into a glass and asking his audience what was in the glass. A little girl said, "Orange juice, stupid." Dyer acknowledged that she was right and said that no matter how hard you squeeze the orange, you will always get orange juice.[18] It is the same with us. No matter how hard we squeeze, the only thing that will come out of us is what is in us, which is our core beliefs about ourselves. We will not be angry unless there is anger in us. We will not be successful unless there is success in us.

I changed destiny by establishing a successful belief system and by building a backlog of successes. Step by step and inch by inch over many years, I became a valuable person in my own mind. Success is a habit, and it is habit-forming.

My 4-Step Formula

In looking back, I realize that my mother and I used four steps to accomplish our goals. With this, I built a success foundation layer-by-layer, year-by-year that is now strong and reliable. This is the four-step success formula:

Success Formula:

1. Determine your goal

2. Do exhaustive research

3. Take action

   - Evaluate

   - Revise

   - Take action again by trial and error.

4. Affirm Success

The 4-Step Formula at West Georgia

When I arrived at West Georgia College, it was clear that their teaching styles did not include any of the styles in which I had learned. My counselor, Dr. Ann Phillips, and

I set to work figuring out what to do so that I could succeed. We did not know it, but we were actually following the success formula that Mom and I had followed.

We plotted, planned, and formed strategy. We first drew up a list of accommodations I would need to graduate: oral testing, readers note takers, etc.

My Formula:

Step 1: Determine Your Goal.

Our goal was clear. Get the accommodations that would allow me to get a college education. Next, we researched the law, and found out what was available for the learning disabled people and people with other handicaps. The Wheelchair Accommodations Form was the only physical handicap form with which Dr. Phillips and I were familiar, so we used it as our model and revised it to meet my needs.

Step 2: Do Exhaustive Research.

This step was ongoing for me. I was continuously researching the best teachers and going around to find the best note takers and readers. Each time Dr. Phillips and I found something we thought would work; we took action on it.

Step 3: Take Action

If something did not work, I tried again. If a teacher said, "No," I went to other teachers until I found one who would help me, if I had sat around bemoaning my failure, waiting for someone to help me, I would never have reached my goal. It was up to me to take the action necessary for my success.

Step 4: Affirm Success.

This occurred whenever I received notice of achieving a small goal or passing a class. To highlight my success, I would paste each "good news letter" on my mirror. It reminded me that I was a successful person. To this day, I have a "power wall" in my office full of photographs, drawings, and other memorabilia that represent my success. I do not think of this as bragging. It is not for other people; it is for me. Whenever I have self-doubt, I look at my wall and remember the exhilarating feeling of being "Player of the Week" or reading my story in the Rockdale County Citizen. That makes it hard to play the "poor little me" game. I am reminded of who I am: a creative, talented individual. I created the "Power Wall" not to remind me of what I have done, but to remind me of what I can do.

Success is Success is Success

I have found that this 4-step success formula works in almost any area of life. Recently, I used it to lose sixty pounds and become fit. One day I looked into the mirror and did not like what I saw. I was an overweight thirty-year-old man. I had little energy and looked older than my age. I thought about my fiancée and the fact that I would probably be in my middle to late thirties by the time we had children. I wanted to participate actively and energetically in their lives. I also wanted to live a long life and see them grow up. These were strong motivations for me to shape up.

My goal was to go from 225 pounds to 165 pounds, and to become physically fit. Step 1 was accomplished; the goal was clear. Next, I did Step 2 by studying health and fitness magazines. From the information I collected, I chose the path of changing my eating habits and adopting a healthier lifestyle rather than going on a severe diet to lose weight. I committed to a fitness routine. To demonstrate my commitment, I joined a gym and paid in advance for a one-year membership. I also committed to spend one hour on the treadmill each morning. These things were great for my body. To exercise my mind at the same time, I decided to listen to educational or motivational tapes or watch educational TV. Step 3, an action plan, was under way. And I did it all.

In this systematic and disciplined way, I not only lost weight and became physically fit, I also changed my perception about aging and eating habits. When I achieved my goal after eight months, I wanted a way to celebrate and affirm this success. That was Step 4. My fiancée suggested that I contact a modeling agency for a photo shoot. I did, and the following picture resulted. My photograph

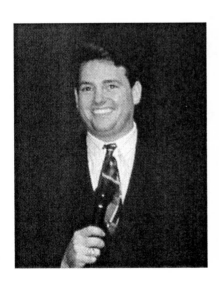
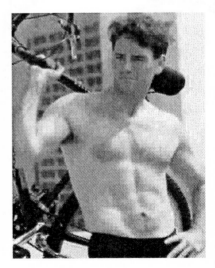

appeared in a national men's hairstyle book. I have no intention of being a model. I only wanted a way to remind myself of my weight loss and fitness success. Upon the birth of my daughter five years later, I was still at my goal weight.

Accept Support

My family made certain that I participated in activities in which I could be successful. With each success, big or small, my value increased in my own eyes.

Professional coaching and other programs can be extremely valuable when you are in the process of internalizing new beliefs, especially new beliefs about success. One of my first glimpses of success was in the SOAR program in middle school. I was as good as anyone in the outdoor activities that made up this program. It was one of the first experiences I had where I achieved success. It felt great.

I definitely wanted to recreate this feeling in other areas of my life, so I went on a search for ways to be successful. Playing football in high school was a major chapter in my success book. Discovering that my friends still liked me when they found out I had a learning disability was another. Anthony Robbins' Firewalk Seminar, where I walked on fire as a metaphor for taking charge of my life by changing my belief systems, was another. Going to see Dr. Ron, the psychologist/hypnotherapist who taught me about visualization, was another.

Today I have several support groups that are vital to my work: my family, the For the Children Foundation, and my friends. In some ways, my story is really the story of the many people who helped me over the years and who were instrumental in my success. To be successful, most people need strong support groups. I found throughout my school days and now in my adult life that people like to feel needed and will gladly help when asked. Support should be a two-way street, in which both people give and receive benefit.

Finding the Meaning in Your Life

Believing in myself got me through the educational system. Since then, I have added another ingredient to success. My first job experience taught me about this important element. As a new graduate just entering the "real world," I had visions of a lifestyle that included fancy cars, expensive clothes and jewelry, and a luxurious home. To me, success meant a lot of money. I quickly found this kind of success. I took great pride in jumping into my 300ZX Twin Turbo Car, tooling along the highway at high speeds, watching heads turn as I passed. I had arrived.

But one morning when my alarm went off, I hit the snooze button and promptly went back to sleep. Several more times the alarm sounded and I continued to cut it off and return to a deep sleep. I never got out of bed that day. When I finally roused myself, I was confused and upset. This behavior was foreign to me. Generally, I am a responsible, hard working, enthusiastic person. When I did go back to my job, I felt almost no enthusiasm or joy. I did not know what was wrong.

To my relief, the answer soon became very clear. I was working for money. Peace of mind, personal satis-faction and a feeling of accomplishment were missing. I lacked a life purpose or mission. I was wandering aimlessly through life, thinking that possessions would satisfy my inner hunger for success. They did not.

I had to ask myself, "If money is not success for me, what is? What makes me happy? What gives me a feeling of satisfaction and accomplishment?"

In college, I had received a ten-week paid internship as a recruiter for the West Georgia Admissions Department. As I thought about my future, I thought back to those college days and the satisfaction I experienced speaking to young people. Recruiting had "accidentally" lead me to speak on learning disabilities.

While recruiting for West Georgia College in a small Georgia town, I had offhandedly mentioned to a counselor that I was learning disabled. He immediately asked if I could come back the next day to speak to his learning disabled students. I had another school to go to the next day so I told him I would not be able to come back. When I reached my motel, my appointment to recruit the following day was canceled. I called the counselor and agreed to return to speak even though I had never spoken publicly about my learning disability before. Although I was ill prepared to speak on the topic of learning disabilities, the group did not seem to notice. Afterward, I recognized from their response that I was making a difference in their lives and I loved doing it. That made me happy.

How could I have forgotten? My life purpose was staring me in the face: I wanted to have a positive impact on the lives of young people and change the educational system.

My sister recently brought a book titled *The Purpose of Your Life* to my attention. The author, Carol Adrienne, offers ten questions that she says will tell you if you are following you life's purpose. She notes that most people

For the Children

cannot answer the questions. In reading the questions, I realized that I had answered all of them when I was determining my life purpose. In fact, my purpose was so clear that my fiancée could also answer the questions about my life.

We draw success to us when our goal is clear. Conversely, no success is possible until we consciously look for and determine our life's purpose.

When your mission becomes clear, the path to the goal begins to unfold naturally. Decisions are easy because you base them on whether or not they support you in reaching your goal. As soon as my mission became clear, the Kroger Company gave me the opportunity to present fifty programs a year under their "Krogering for Kids" program. I was excited to be doing what I love to do, and at the same time, offering value to others. I felt that if I truly offered service to others, the money would follow. It did. Eventually, Kroger hired me to represent them in giving seventy school talks per year. I was now doing what I love and supporting myself by doing it. When the alarm sounds at 4:00 a.m. on a day that I am to give an out of town talk; I bounce out of bed with excitement and anticipation, eager to begin the new day.

When you know your life's purpose and are acting in accordance with it, life is like floating down a river to success. It is easy as long as you do not try to "push the river" or control it. Swim with the current. Be flexible. When I veer off the path away from my mission, I immediately feel the ramifications and my life is no longer running smoothly. I recognize the problem, correct it, and continue on my path. Life is a series of corrections.

Ignore the Nay-sayers

When you get serious about your goal, you cannot listen to nay-sayers. Listen only to those who support you in reaching the goal. Along the way to weight loss and physical fitness, some people said to me, "You look fine the way you are." Others said, "Adults always gain weight as they grow older." After losing the weight, several people said in a reproachful tone, "You look like a boy." These people meant well, but if I had listened to them, I would have allowed others to direct my life. No one knows better than I do about what gives me happiness and fulfillment. I have to be true to myself.

Just before I got my college degree, someone who said it could not be done almost stopped me. My last semester, I pre-registered for an Art History class that was required for my degree. The class was canceled, leaving eight of us without a credit we needed to receive our degrees. I immediately went to the chairman of my department, explained the situation, told him I had a job waiting for me, and asked to be allowed to substitute another class for Art History.

He said, "No." In fact, he ended our meeting with, "See you back here next fall." I was angry, but I knew that being a victim would not change my circumstances. I revved up my, "blue collar", action mode. I marched into the office of the Dean of Arts and Sciences and explained my dilemma.

"Sure," he said, "go ahead and make the substitution."

I received my degree. Strangely, I was the only one of the eight in my circumstance who went to bat for myself and graduated on schedule. Thank God for mother's training which taught me to never accept "No" as a final answer.

Find Inspiration

Christopher Reeves inspires me. He may be a paraplegic, but he has said many times that he is blessed. Since his accident, he has worked tirelessly to improve the quality of life for other paralyzed individuals. Some day, many that cannot walk today may walk because of his efforts. He has a life purpose, one that has given him the will to live.

Every day read or listen to inspiring books. Incorporate the success message into your life and actions. When Chicken Soup for the Soul was first published, I read it repeatedly and was inspired each time. I would call my mom and read her stories from the book, even as poorly as I read. Each time I called, she had to tell me if she was ready for another story. She would say, "No, Rob, today is not the day for a story. I cannot cry today because I have to go somewhere this afternoon." This did not dampen my enthusiasm for Chicken Soup for the Soul or for the inspiration and uplift it gave me.

Several other things have been important in my success, especially fun and laughter. Life does not have to be a struggle. Struggle or ease; it is all in you perception. Laughter makes you feel happier. Studies have shown that it enhances health. Recreate the wonder and happiness of a young child.

Visualization: Your Most Powerful Tool

I have been using visualization to reach my goals since high school when Dr. Ron helped me learn to lift weights using this technique. I use it in business, finances, success with speaking, and any number of other areas. Some time ago, I made the decision to use it for something fun.

I am not a big sports fan, but I love the Atlanta Braves. I thought to myself, 'If you could talk to any of the Braves, who would it be?' I decided it would be Greg Maddux. I did not know him at all, but I thought it would be fun to speak with him. I decided to use a combination of visualization and my success formula.

First I had to decide what I wanted. I wanted to talk to Greg Maddux. Second, I had to do extensive research and get educated on the subject. I went on the Internet and found out all about Greg Maddux. He lives in Las Vegas with his wife and kids and he loves golf. He likes to play in the morning and spends afternoon with his family. On the Braves web page, up pops a picture of Greg, which is important in my visualization. I pulled that picture off the Internet and laminated it. I then put it up on my bathroom mirror so it was the first thing I saw each morning.

The key to visualization is that you are going to get what you think about all day. If I want to meet Greg Maddux, I need to see him every day. After a few mornings of this, I started having a conversation with Greg in my mind. I started to think what I would talk to him about: golf and Las Vegas. Over the next month, I built up about an hour-long conversation with Greg. Before I knew it, I began to believe I was going to meet Greg Maddux. I started telling people "I am going to meet Greg Maddux"

One day I was telling a man and he said, "Well, I know Greg Maddux."

"Wait a minute. You know him?" I said

"Sure. How would you like to play golf with him?"

I said, "That is what I have been visualizing."He

explained that the John Smoltz's Celebrity Amateur Tournament was coming up and Greg Maddux would be there. It cost $1,000 to play and he had already paid for himself. Then, he offered to let me play in his place. I was going to play golf with Greg Maddux and I did not even have to pay.

I was so excited the day of the tournament. I drove to the Atlanta Country Club and pulled in past all the fancy cars. I was thinking, 'This is a good visualization.' I found my parking space, grabbed my clubs and walked-up to the front of the clubhouse. Standing there to meet me was John Smoltz. He said, "Here Rob, let me take those clubs for you. We will put them in the cart. You will be teeing off from the sixth tee. Go on into the clubhouse. We have some breakfast for you."

The only problem was, John was not my visualization and so I did not know what to do. So I said, "AAHHHHH-HHH." I was star struck and fear struck. I just made noises and went in. I was so early; there was no one else there. I did what I always do when something good happens. I called my mother. I went back to the car and whipped out the cell phone. I started telling her about my visualization and how I was going to meet Greg Maddux and I had already met John Smoltz. This was going to be a great day.

Suddenly, I looked around and realized it was 8:00 am. I went back into the clubhouse and sure enough, the entire room was full. Now I was the last person in line. I was thinking I was not hungry and maybe I would go back to the car and call Mom back. I could talk to her until tee time.

I was walking out the front door of the clubhouse and there he was. Greg Maddux! He was walking straight towards me. I thought, 'Is that really him? Surely he is not my height.' He walked by me and someone stopped him to talk. I turned to him and put out my hand. I said, "Hi Greg, my name is Rob Langston and I am heading out to Vegas in two weeks with my fiancée. I wondered if you could recommend a golf course?" I had planned this trip six months earlier.

He said, "Sure, you have to play Shadow Creek." And then he turned around and walked on. I said to myself, 'Wait a minute. I have an hour with you!' The conversation that I had visualized lasted much longer.

I went through the line and got my food. When I scanned the room for a place to sit, there was one seat left. It was next to Greg Maddux. I made eye contact with him and he gave me a wave. I said to myself, 'I do not believe this.' I walked over, sat down, and looked up to see a sign that explained why the seat was empty. I was at the Players' Table.

Smoltz and all the other important guys were sitting there. I had not visualized any of them. Greg and I sat there for the entire meal. I monopolized him, talking about everything I had visualized. It lasted about an hour and it was the most fun I had ever had.

I did not play golf with him, but I did talk to him again. After the tournament John Smoltz grabbed me by the shoulder and said, "I heard you talking to Greg about playing golf in Vegas. You had better run and catch up to him because Shadow Creek is owned by the Mirage Hotel and they only let a handful of people play that course."

I caught up with Greg and said, "John told me you may need to get a tee time for me out there."

He said, "Okay, here is my home phone number. Give me a call when you get out there." I had done Step #3 and

Step #4 of the formula for success. I had certainly taken action. I was affirming success like crazy.

Understand this. If I had gone up to Greg Maddux on the street and said, "Hi Greg, my name is Rob Langston. Give me your home phone number so I can get a tee time from you?" He would have run from me like I was a stalker.

Also, understand that you will see a person's best face when they are doing for others. We were at a charity golf tournament to raise money to support a hospital and Greg was in the giving spirit. He was probably kinder to me than he might otherwise have been because of the circumstance.

The next day I took a photograph of the entire team and placed it on my mirror. I have since met or played golf with almost every single member of the Atlanta Braves.

Visualization works. I did not make it up. It has been around forever and it has worked. The only question is: How soon will you start making it work for you?

If you use the techniques I have described in this book, you will have success. When you do, I challenge you to do something with it! I challenge you to do something for someone else with it. That is what our world needs.

Whether you are a child in the educational system or an adult in the "real world," it is up to you to create your own success. Believe in yourself. Love what you do. Decide what you want, conduct exhaustive research on your goal, take action, and affirm your victories. Make this a good life. Strengthen your commitment and focus. You will pull in others to help you reach your goal. Success is in your hands.[19]

End Notes

1   Dr. Harold Levinson, a world-renowned psychiatrist and neurologist, began his pioneering research on dyslexia 35 years ago within the New York City Board of Education.

2   Fire walking demonstrates how your thoughts impact everything else in your life. Thoughts change brain chemistry, and that results in an alteration of body chemistry as well. Firewalkers are instructed to pay close attention to their thoughts, since those very thoughts are the way in which we create our own realities. Positive thinkers literally live in a different chemical environment than negative thinkers.

3   Offered by the Nation Library Service of the Library of Congress. See www.LOC.gov

4   The International Dyslexia Association

5   The Dyslexia Institute website at www.Dyslexia-inst.org.uk

6   The Merriam-Webster Dictionary, Merriam Webster Inc., Springfield, MA, 1999.

7   Dyer, Wayne. Improve Your Life Using the Wisdom of Ages, Hay House Inc. 1998

8   Ibid

9   Interview: Dr. Ann Phillips, Ph. D, L. P. C. Coordinator of Disabled Student Services, State University of West Georgia.

10 Daniel P. Hallahan and James M. Kauffman,
Exceptional Learners, 8th ed.,
Allyn and Bacon, Inc., 1999.

11 Office of Special Education Programs Office of
Special Education and Rehabilitative Services U.S.
Department of Education Washington, DC 20202.
The Individuals with Disabilities Education Act
Amendments of 1997 Public Law 105-17, were
signed by the President on June 4, 1997. The Final
IDEA '97 Regulations were released on Friday,
March 12, 1999.

12 We strive to provide leadership and support to
members by providing input into the policies and
practices in Georgia which impact the quality of
education and by providing support to the
professionals who serve the students of Georgia

13 Jastak Associates, Inc.: The Wide Range
Achievement Test (WRAT) is a brief achievement
test measuring reading recognition, spelling, and
arithmetic computation. There are two levels; level I
is normed for children ages 5 to 11; level II is the
norm for children aged 12 through adults aged 64.

14 Formal academic education is provided in some
prisons at several levels. Illiteracy, defined as
performance at less than the fourth-grade level,
prevails among about 30% of those offenders
admitted to prison. Remedying this condition is one
of the basic and challenging tasks of correctional
education. Prisoners are often pathetically pleased
when they learn to read letters from home and to
write them. (Tappan, 1960, p. 690)

15 Dr. Howard Gardner, <u>Frames of Mind: The Theory of Multiple Intelligences</u>, 10th edition, Basic Books, 1993.

16 Federation of Families for Children's Mental Health Alexandria, Virginia 22314 www.ffcmh.org ffcmh@ffcmh.org

A National parent-run non-profit organization focused on the needs of children and youth with emotional, behavioral or mental disorders and their families.

17 IDEA: http://www.ideapractices.org/law/index.php

18 Dyer, Wayne. <u>Improve Your Life Using the Wisdom of Ages</u>, Hay House Inc. 1998

19 Colin Rose and Malcolm J. Nicholl. <u>Accelerated Learning For the 21st Century: a Six Step Plan to Unlock Your Master Mind</u>, Dimensions, 1998.

Bibliography

Canfield, Jack and Mark Victor Hansen. <u>Chicken Soup for the Soul: 101 Stories to Open the Heart and Rekindle the Spirit</u>. Health Communications, Inc. 2001.

Smith, Donn O. State of Georgia, Department of Corrections.

Dyer, Wayne. <u>Improve Your Life Using the Wisdom of Ages</u>. New York: Hays House, Inc., 1998.

Dyslexia Institute. http://www.dyslexia-inst.org.uk

Federation of Families for Children's Mental Health Alexandria. www.ffcmh.org ffcmh@ffcmh.org

Gardner, Dr. Howard. <u>Frames of Mind: The Theory of Multiple Intelligences</u>, 10th edition. New York: Basic Books, 1993.

Hallahan, Daniel P. and James M. Kauffman, <u>Exceptional Learners</u>, 8th ed.Boston:, Allyn and Bacon, Inc., 1999.

IDEA. The Individuals with Disabilities Education Act Amendments of 1997 Public Law 105-17. : http://www.ideapractices.org/law/index.php

International Dyslexia Association. http://www.interdys.org/index.jsp

<u>International Who's Who of Entrepreneurs</u>, Gibralter Publishing, Inc., 414 Bell Fork Road, Jacksonville, North Carolina 28541

Jastak, J. F., & Jastak, S. Wide range interest-opinion test. Wilmington, DE: 1979.

Levinaon, Dr. Harold. Center for Learning Disabilities. http://www.dyslexiaonline.com

Levinaon, Dr. Harold. A Solution to the Riddle - Dyslexia. London: Stonebridge Publishing, Ltd. 2000.

Merriam-Webster Third New International Dictionary, 3rd edition. Merriam Webster, Inc., Springfield, MA, 1999.

Phillips, Dr. Ann, Ph.D., L.P.C., Coordinator of Disabled Student Services, State University of West Georgia.

Robbins, Anthony. Tony Robbins Seminars, Robbins Research International, Inc. http://www.robbinsresearch.com

Rose, Colin and Malcolm J. Nicholl. Accelerated Learning For the 21st Century: a Six Step Plan to Unlock Your Master Mind, Dimensions, 1998.

Tappan, 1960, http://www.firewalking.com

Printed in the United States
1297400001B/172-249